RECOMBINANT ANTIBODIES

RECOMBINANT ANTIBODIES

Frank Breitling, Stefan Dübel

A JOHN WILEY & SONS, INC. and SPEKTRUM AKADEMISCHER VERLAG CO-PUBLICATION

WILEY New York · Chichester · Weinheim · Brisbane · Singapore · Toronto

Heidelberg · Berlin

Original title: Rekombinante Antikörper
Translated from German by Tatiana Kassessinoff

German edition
© 1998 by Spektrum Akademischer Verlag

English edition
© 1999 jointly by John Wiley & Sons, Inc. and Spektrum Akademischer Verlag

John Wiley & Sons, Inc
605 Third Avenue
New York, NY 10158-0012
USA

Spektrum Akademischer Verlag
Vangerowstrasse 20
D-69115 Heidelberg
Germany

Telephone: (212) 850-6000

Telephone: 49 6221 91260

Address all inquiries to John Wiley & Sons, Inc.

While the authors, editors and publisher believe that drug selection and dosage and the specificati-
on and usage of equipment and devices, as set forth in this book, are in accord with current
recommendations and practice at the time of publication, they accept no legal responsibility for
any errors or omissions, and make no warranty, expressed or implied, with respect to material
contained herein. In view of ongoing research, equipment modifications, changes in governmental
regulations and the constant flow of information relating to drug therapy, drug reactions, and the
use of equipment and devices, the reader is urged to review and evaluate the information provided
in the package insert or instructions for each drug, piece of equipment, or device for, among other
things, any changes in instructions or indication of dosage or usage and for added warnings and
precautions.

Library of Congress Cataloging-in-Publication Data

Recombinant antibodies / edited by Stefan Dübel, Frank Breitling.
     p. cm.
  Includes bibliographical references and index.
  ISBN 0-471-17847-0
    1. Recombinant antibodies. I. Dübel, Stefan. II. Breitling, Frank.
QR186.87.R43   1999
616.07'98--dc21   99-14610
                                                CIP

Die Deutsche Bibliothek – CIP-Einheitsaufnahme

Breitling, Frank:
Recombinant antibodies / Frank Breitling ; Stefan Dübel. New York ;
Chichester ; Weinheim ; Brisbane ; Singapore ; Toronto : Wiley ;
Heidelberg ; Berlin : Spektrum, Akad. Verl., 1999
  Dt. Ausg. u.d.T.: Breitling, Frank: Rekombinante Antikörper
  ISBN 0-471-17847-0

The text of this book is printed on acid-free paper.

Printed in the United States of America.
10 9 8 7 6 5 4 3 2 1

Contents

Preface

The field of recombinant antibodies is barely ten years old and has already attracted a large number of scientists and is becoming routine in more laboratories. The goal is usually the production of human monoclonal antibodies for therapy and diagnosis - a goal that was often not attainable before.

This books is aimed at interested students, technical assistants and scientists that have come into contact with this field for the first time. We have endeavored to write it in such a way that only a little forehand knowledge is needed to fully understand it. We have also continually tried to answer concrete questions that arise in the laboratory routine or, at least, to provide the route to these answers through the extensive bibliography of original references.

The first two chapters define the role of the immune system as the teacher of genetic engineers. All the principles used in the construction of and the search for recombinant antibodies are derived from examples in the human body. Recombinant antibody technology is meanwhile able to do more than the immune system. This offers a way to produce antibodies that the immune system is unable to, for example, antibodies against toxins or strongly pathogenic antigens.

Recombinant technology also offers a subsequent important innovation in addition to the generation of antibodies that previously could not be produced. The genetic fusion to proteins with different functions opens new avenues for the use of antibodies in research, diagnosis and therapy. Recombinant antibodies promise to be of great use in medical applications, especially in tumor therapy. These new possibilities are the subject of the third chapter. The fundamental principles of recombinant antibody technology were developed within a few years. Initially, the approach appeared to be straightforward and simple. The technical difficulties associated with the construction and especially the production and use of recombinant antibodies only became clear with time. This book attempts to point out these problems and to provide potential solutions. As such, we would like to help newcomers circumvent some traps that the authors were not spared. Many such suggestions are found in the fourth chapter.

At this point we would especially like to thank Gerd Moldenhauer, Roland Kontermann, Martin Welschof, Eva Schüßler, Eckard Fuchs and Susanne Rondot for whose critiques were vital to this book, and Uschi Loos from the Spektrum Akademischer Verlag for her many suggestions and her patience. Prof. Ekkehard Bautz and Prof. Melvyn Little have also strongly supported us with their understanding of this extensive work and their patience. We also thank Ingrid Hermes, Iris Klewinghaus and Iris Queitsch whose work in the laboratory liberated us to work on the book. Special thanks go to our families for their understanding and support.

Frank Breitling
Stefan Dübel

Chapter 1
Background

This book is about recombinant antibodies. A complete overview of the immune system would exceed the scope of this book and, therefore, the reader is advised to consult relevant textbooks such as the outstanding *Immunology* by Charles Janeway and Paul Travers (1997). Individual aspects of the humoral immune response are highlighted, however, to allow a comparison between our immune system and recombinant techniques. In this way, we would like to convey a feeling for the fascinating solutions that the immune system has developed during millions of years of evolution. This book shows how the principles that govern the humoral immune response were adapted to the test tube - by genetic engineers inspired from evolution.

1.1 How the Body Manufactures Antibodies

1.1.1 THE CHANCE COMBINATION OF PEPTIDE BUILDING BLOCKS LEADS TO A VAST VARIETY OF ANTIBODIES

Antibodies are a component of the immune system, which constitutes a versatile defense system of the body against intruders. The main purpose of antibodies is to bind pathogens specifically and thereby mark them for the immune system.

How can an organism manage to raise a specific antibody against practically every foreign substance? How can it recognize almost all potential "enemy" *antigens*? Humans achieve this through a huge arsenal of antibodies with different binding specificities. For the human body, maintaining an autonomous gene for each of the estimated more than 10^8 different antibodies would be far too extravagant. The resulting amount of necessary information would exceed the capacity of the genome. Vertebrates (only they possess antibodies) have solved this problem with the help of an elegant trick. In the same way that millions of different houses can be built with only a few types of standard bricks, "standard" polypeptide building blocks are linked together to form

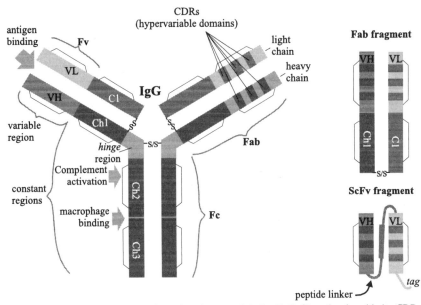

Fig. 1.1. Schematic representation of an immunoglobulin G (IgG) molecule with its CDRs: complementarity-determining-regions; antigen-binding frangments. C1, Ch1 to Ch3: constant regions; VL: variable region of the light chain; VH: variable region of the heavy chain; peptide linker: joins the VH and the VL; *tag*: C-terminal extension to change the biochemical properties of the fusion protein; S/S: disulfide bridge.

module-based antibodies. As such, only a few hundred of these polypeptide building blocks need to be encoded in the genome. A few (large) building blocks code for the constant domains of an antibody, thereby determining its effector functions, which are to ensure the transfer of messages to the immune system. However, the *antigen*-binding specificity of an antibody is mediated by only a small part of the total molecule: the *variable regions* (Fig. 1.1). These are made up of two to three different modules that are put together in different ways in each cell during the process of B-lymphocyte differentiation. Besides the recombination of these gene fragments, random mechanisms exist that can arbitrarily insert short, new sequences at the fusion points of various gene fragments. The variety of possible structures is increased further by another trick, which comprises the combination of two, independent protein chains (the "light" and "heavy" antibody chains) into one protein complex (Figs. 1.1 and 1.2). Both protein elements can then contribute to antigen binding.

1.1.2 THE SPECIFICITY OF ANTIGEN BINDING IS DETERMINED BY THE HYPERVARIABLE DOMAINS

When a comparison is made between antibody sequences, three peptide sequences of 5 to 15 amino acids within each variable region stand out, which can contain a variety of different peptide sequences (reviewed in Kabat et al., 1987). Though distributed over the length of the antibody sequence, in the final, folded protein, these *hypervariable regions* are found together on an outer

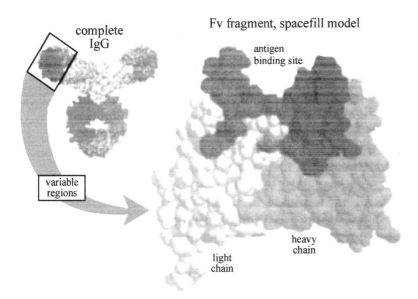

complete
IgG

Fv fragment, spacefill model

antigen
binding site

variable
regions

heavy
chain

light
chain

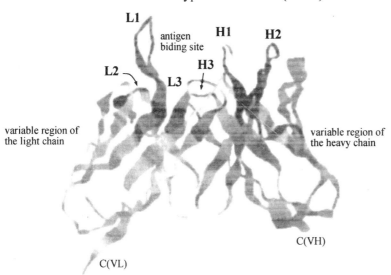

Cα atom framework: hypervariable areas (CDRs)

L1

antigen
biding site

H1   H2

L2

H3

L3

variable region of
the light chain

variable region of
the heavy chain

C(VH)

C(VL)

Fig. 1.2. The Fv fragment is the portion of an antibody that is responsible for the antigen specificity. **Top**: An IgG molecule (*left*) contains two Fv fragments (*right*) (also shown enlarged). The hypervariable areas (or CDRs) responsible for contact with the antigen are darkly shaded. **Bottom**: Cα ribbon representation that clarifies the framework of β-sheet structures, which are responsible for the extraordinary stabilty of antibody molecules. The contact site with the antigen is formed from six peptide loops, three from each of the heavy and light chains (H1 to H3, L1 to L3). The models are based on coordinates kindly made available by R. Kontermann and A. Martin.

surface (Fig. 1.2). In total, six of these hypervariable regions (three from each of the light and heavy chains) represent the actual contact point of the antibody with an antigen. These regions are also called *complementarity-determining regions* (CDRs) because they form a structure that is complementary to the antigen. The role of the remaining part of the variable region is to stabilize the spatial structure of the hypervariable domain. This occurs by virtue of the highly rigid β-sheet structure of the framework.

1.1.3 THE CONSTANT REGIONS STABILIZE THE ANTIBODY MOLECULE

The two variable domains of the light and heavy chains form a common antigen-binding site. The coupling of these domains alone, however, usually is relatively weak ($K_d \sim 10^{-6}$ mol). Additional bonds are necessary to stabilize the antibody molecule. These bonds are provided by the *constant regions* that make up a large part of the overall molecule. One (sometimes several) disulfide bridge between the constant regions of the light and heavy chains enables their covalent coupling. Further disulfide bridges link the constant regions of the heavy chains into a dimer resulting in two identical antigen-binding sites. In certain classes of antibodies, even more of these molecular complexes are bound together (an IgA molecule has four to six antigen-binding sites, an IgM molecule has ten).

1.1.4 THE CONSTANT REGIONS MEDIATE THE EFFECTOR FUNCTIONS

Only in a few special cases does an antibody practice its protective function by itself. Neutralizing antibodies exist against bacterial toxins as do antibodies that prevent the viral invasion of target cells. The humoral system is most effective through its activation of the rest of the immune system. This activation is mediated by the constant regions, whereas the variable domains bind and thereby mark the target.

Various constant regions can mediate a whole range of different biological effects. An allergic reaction, for example, follows IgE binding, whereas IgM binding can lead to the activation of the complement system. The modular design of the molecule also allows for an exchange of the constant regions (a class switch) while retaining antigen specificity. According to the requirement, the immune system can thus react in a very flexible way during the development of the immune response.

1.1.5 ANTIBODY BINDING IMPROVES DURING AN IMMUNE RESPONSE

It has long been known that the immune response can improve over time. As such, certain diseases are contracted only once, and thereafter the body is protected against these germs or said to be "immune". This improvement has also been shown for individual antibodies. When a mouse is immunized with a small antigen, a *hapten*, the subsequently generated antibodies (the immunoglobulins) bind relatively weakly to the antigen at first. If, after some

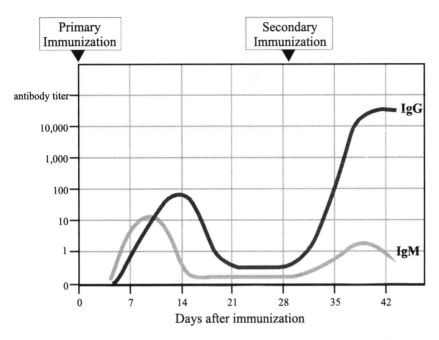

Fig. 1.3. Time course of the primary and secondary immune response. In a typical immune response, the reaction resulting from a second immunization is faster, stronger, and predominantly through IgG. The reasons for this improved response are illustrated in Figures 1.4 and 1.5.

time, the immunization is repeated, the antibodies then generated bind this antigen much better (Fig. 1.3). Over time, an *affinity maturation* occurs (Janeway and Travers, 1997).

1.1.6 B-LYMPHOCYTES ARE EXPANDED THROUGH CLONAL SELECTION

Recent studies have elucidated the mechanisms leading to *affinity maturation*. An antigen (e.g., a "flu" virus) is faced with an estimated repertoire of more than 10^8 different antibodies. Each antibody is originally formed from a single B-lymphocyte, in whose nucleus a random, genetic combination occurred for the above mentioned polypeptide module of the antibody. Each specific antibody from the repertoire is presented on the surface of "its" B-lymphocyte while circulating through the body (Fig. 1.4). Only a few of the B-lymphocytes from this repertoire actually carry antibodies, directed against a certain antigen, on their surface. Binding to this antigen triggers these cells to divide. In this way, the proportion of this special B-lymphocyte *clone* is significantly expanded with respect to the total population. A *clonal selection* occurs. Some of these B-lymphocytes develop further into antibody-secreting plasma cells. With the help of alternate splicing of the antibody mRNA, the plasma cell switches from membrane-bound antibodies (mIg) to a form that can be secreted (Ig). Other B-lymphocytes from the expanded clone once again

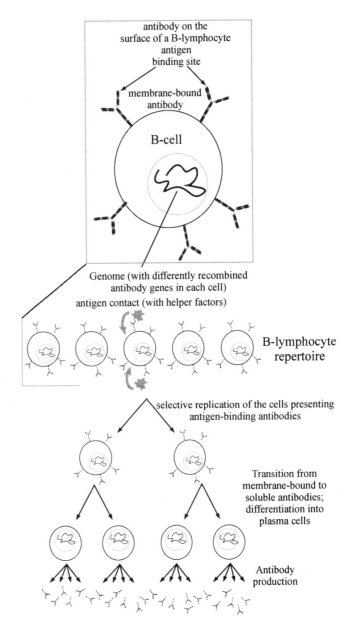

Fig. 1.4. Clonal selection: Development of the primary immune response. A large repertoire of B-lymphocytes circulate in the blood that have each conducted different gene rearragements. Each B-lymphocyte presents "its" specific antibody on its surface. Antibody-mediated contact with an antigen-presenting cell, activates a growth program in this B-lymphocyte. The B-lymphocyte greatly replicates itself (clonal selection). A proportion of its descendants differentiate into plasma cells. These then secrete large amounts of the selected antibody.

recombine their genomic DNA, thereby fusing the gene coding for another constant chain to the selected variable gene. This process is called an *isotype exchange* or class switch.

1.1.7 ONLY THOSE MEMORY CELLS SURVIVE THAT CODE FOR HIGHER AFFINITY ANTIBODIES

About one week after stimulation with an antigen, the plasma cells have produced a large number of antibodies. This results in an excess of antibodies in relation to the antigen (the "flu" virus, for example), which is thereby eliminated. Around this time, *germinal centers* arise in the lymph nodes each originating from a few fast dividing B-lymphocytes. In these cells the genes for the rearranged, variable antibody domains (and only these genes!) are subjected to an extremely high mutation rate. It is estimated that through *somatic hypermutation* about 1 in 10^3 base pairs are mutated, for each cell division. This is a billionfold increase over the normal mutation rate.

Very few of these mutations code for an antibody with improved affinity for the antigen. How do these improved binding variants manage to dominate? In the germinal centers, antibody-presenting B-lymphocytes compete with each other for binding to the antigen-presenting *follicular dendritic cells*. This binding is a matter of survival for the B-lymphocytes, which would otherwise carry out a programmed cell death, that is, die through the process of *apoptosis*. The cells not only compete with each other for the scarce, dendritic cell-presented antigens. Equally important, is the competition with the many, already generated, soluble antibodies. Thus, only those B-lymphocytes that present antibodies with superior binding properties have a chance to bind antigen, a process essential for their survival. Out of these surviving B-lymphocytes the *memory cells* eventually develop, in which the mutations that led to improved binding not only merely survived, but superseded the original ancestral antibody gene. In a second immune response, these memory cells ensure that the antigen is eliminated much faster. An *affinity maturation* has taken place (Fig. 1.5).

1.1.8 EVOLUTION INVENTED ANTIBODY ENGINEERING MILLIONS OF YEARS AGO

Evolution invented the humoral immune system in higher vertebrates millions of years ago. This formidable defense is governed by 3 simple principles:
-   the chance combination of peptide building blocks
-   the clonal selection of specific antibodies together with their corresponding B-lymphocytes and finally
-   affinity maturation of antibodies.

Thus millions of different antibodies are generated, mutated and selected. Throughout life in each individual, the humoral immune system evolves in response to an antigenic challenge. The result of this individual evolution is constantly improved antibodies, and this is precisely what genetic engineers attempt to do with recombinant antibodies in the test tube.

Other applications are influenced by these principles as well. With all standard vaccination protocols the individual immunizations are conducted a minimum of four weeks apart. This roughly represents the time span needed for affinity maturation, that is, the process of memory cell formation.

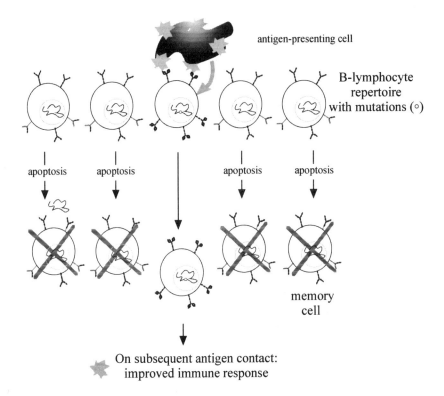

antigen-presenting cell

B-lymphocyte
repertoire
with mutations (○)

apoptosis   apoptosis   apoptosis   apoptosis

memory
cell

On subsequent antigen contact:
improved immune response

Fig. 1.5. Memory cells provide for the improvement of the antibody and an accelerated secondary immune response. They are descendents of B-lymphocytes that compete for the antigen in the germinal centres, where the variable genes simultaneously mutate at a billion fold increased rate. Out of these only those cells survive that remain in contact with the antigen-presenting folicular dendritic cells, which selects for antibodies with higher affinity for the antigen. Therefore, those mutations will superscale the original antibody gene leading to antibodies with an improved affinity for the antigen.

1.2 Antibody Production: Established Methods and New Approaches

1.2.1 ANTIBODIES ARE WIDELY USED IN RESEARCH AND DIAGNOSIS

For several decades antibodies have been indispensible in research and diagnosis due to their specific binding properties and high stability. From the work of Emil Behring and Shibasaburo Kitasato over a century ago, it has been known that specific binding molecules could be acquired from blood (Fig. 1.6). Since then antibodies with a particular specificity are produced by the immunization of laboratory animals with an antigen. A few weeks after immunization the desired antibodies are detected in the animal's serum. Human antibodies can also be produced by this method. However inherently, the scope of this kind of immunization is very limited.

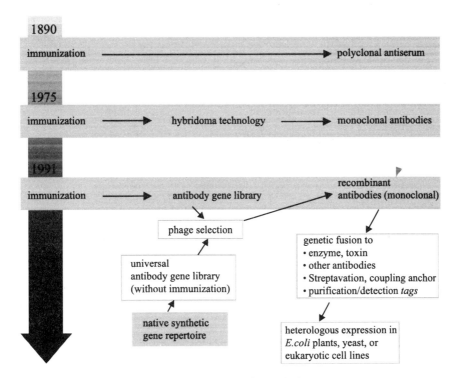

Fig. 1.6.   Historic development of the antibody production methods.

1.2.2 ANTISERA CONTAIN POLYCLONAL ANTIBODIES

Antisera obtained by immunization always contain a *mixture* of antibody proteins with different binding specificities. In the main, the majority of these antibodies do not bind the antigen at all, they were already present before the immunization.

The newly formed antibodies usually represent a mixture of different antigen-specific antibodies. They result from the challenge with large biomolecules used for the immunization, which can accommodate many surface *epitopes* (Fig. 1.7). An epitope is defined as that region of an antigen that actually contacts the antibody. Therefore, many different antibodies are usually generated in the blood in response towards different epitopes of the same antigen. Thus, the term *polyclonal antibody* reflects the action of many different B-lymphocyte clones that secrete their individual antigen- specific antibodies into the blood.

1.2.3 IMMORTAL B-LYMPHOCYTES PRODUCE MONOCLONAL ANTIBODIES

A new method known as the *hybridoma technique* was developed by Köhler and Milstein in 1975.

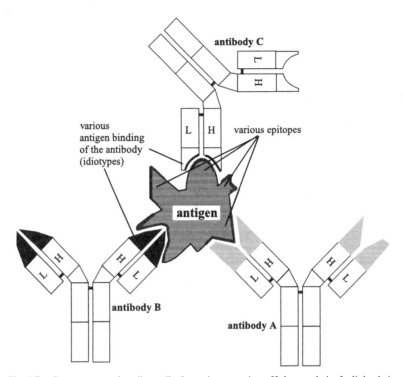

Fig. 1.7. Some terms to describe antibody–antigen reactions. H: heavy chain; L: light chain.

Identical to the generation of polyclonal antibodies, it requires the initial immunization of a laboratory animal (usually a mouse or rat). The resulting antibodies, however, are not obtained directly from the blood serum. Instead the activated B-lymphocytes (precursors of the antibody-producing cells) are isolated from the spleen. Because of its individual gene arrangement, each B-lymphocyte produces antibodies with a single binding affinity (see above). The expanded B-lymphocyte, the B-lymphocyte clone, would then produce monospecific antibodies with this same binding specificity. However, B-lymphocytes rapidly die in cell culture. Therefore, Köhler and Milstein fused the B-lymphocytes with plasmacytoma cells, descendants of a plasma-cell-tumor. The resulting *hybridoma cells* possess the properties of both fusion partners. They are immortal cancer cells that produce an antibody coded for by the B-lymphocyte partner (Köhler and Milstein, 1975). The descendants of a single hybridoma cell (i.e., its clones) produce antibodies with a single defined specificity. These antibodies are therefore called *monoclonal antibodies* (Fig. 1.8). With this technique, which was awarded the Nobel prize, in principle unlimited quantities of a monospecific antibody could be produced for the first time from the immortalized cells. A disadvantage of this method, however, is the labor-intensive procedure needed for the selection of the desired antibody-producing clone from thousands of hybridomas that manufacture irrelevant antibodies.

A good methodological overview of the "classical" techniques of antibody production is available in the volume by Liddell and Weeks (1996) from the same Focus series.

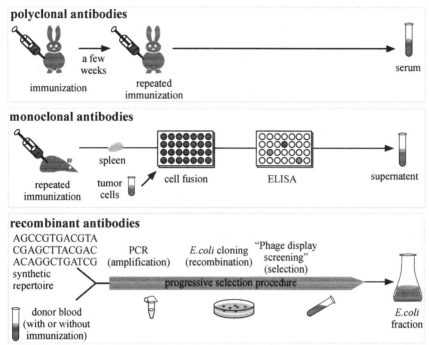

Fig. 1.8. Schematic summary of the different antibody production methods. ELISA: enzyme-linked immunosorbent assay; PCR: polymerase chain reaction.

1.2.4 RECOMBINANT ANTIBODIES ARE GENETICALLY ENGINEERED ANTIBODY FRAGMENTS

With the construction of recombinant antibodies, a third approach for the production of antibodies was recently developed. The antibodies are no longer produced in a laboratory animal (or a human subject), but in bacteria or in cell cultures, *in vitro*. The focus of attention is the antigen-binding portion of the antibody. In order to obtain higher yields, the rest of the antibody molecule is usually relinquished. These fragments can no longer perform all the functions of a naturally produced antibody. They can, however, be fused with enzymes or other antibodies with comparative ease. In this way, recombinant antibodies acquire a completely new set of properties.

Given the numerous possibilities of recombination with other gene fragments, the genetically engineered "recombinant antibodies" are exclusively defined on the basis of the antigen specificity.

1.2.5 Fv FRAGMENTS ARE THE SMALLEST ANTIGEN-BINDING UNITS

For many applications, the smallest possible antigen-binding unit is required. Before the development of recombinant technology, only the *Fab fragments*, created from the protease digestion of normal antibodies, were of practical use (Fig. 1.1). A Fab fragment is made up of the variable regions of both chains stabilized by the adjacent constant domains. Very similar *Fab fragments* can be produced with the use of recombinant methods. However, the smallest molecule that still retains the total antigen-binding site is made up of only the variable regions of the light and heavy chains (see *VL* and *VH* in Figs. 1.1 and 1.2). Similar to Fc (constant region fragments) and Fab (antigen-binding region fragments), these fragments are called Fv (variable region fragments). Such Fv fragments must be stabilized because they are no longer covalently coupled through the cysteines in the constant regions. This is usually done with a *peptide link* that joins the variable domains to a single-chain Fv fragment (= scFv fragment, scFv antibody, Fig. 1.1.)

1.2.6 WHY RECOMBINANT ANTIBODIES?

What is the motivation behind the search for new ways to produce antibodies? The evolution of the immune system has provided a nearly inexhaustible potential for the manufacture of specific binding molecules. This potential is already exploited through the production of polyclonal antisera or monoclonal hybridoma cell lines. What could recombinant antibodies accomplish further?

1.2.6.1 Recombinant Antibodies Can Be Obtained *In Vitro*

In contrast to all the other methods, recombinant antibodies are obtained from a bacterial host that is completely *independent* of a vertebrate. Therefore, the selection of specific antibodies in the test tube avoids possible contamination with AIDS, hepatitis or BSE, a risk always present when human or animal products are used. These recombinant antibodies are, of course, also monoclonal because they originate from a single (bacterial) cell. Just like hybridoma cells, bacterial cells offer the benefits of both immortality and antibodies with a defined epitope specificity. Moreover, bacterial clones are usually simpler and cheaper than the corresponding hybridoma cell clones in terms of handling, culture, analysis, and storage. More important however, is the fact that the entire technology of *E. coli* genetics is available for use in the analysis and modification of these clones. Consequently, sequencing and countless modifications are simplified, or even, for the first time, actually feasible. In this way, antibody fragments can be "humanized" or fused to heterologous genes to form chimeric molecules that exhibit new functions (discussed further in Section 2.3 and Chapter 3).

1.2.6.2 Recombinant Antibodies Can Be Of Human Origin

Currently, recombinant antibodies can be produced without the need for a prior immunization by using *E. coli* genetic libraries, thereby reducing animal experimentation (see also Section 2.2). Most of all, it allows for the production of *human* antibodies *in vitro,* usually a very difficult task with all the other alternative techniques at hand.

Polyclonal sera from immunized humans are expensive and dangerous, highlighted by the fact that numerous patients contracted AIDS or hepatitis from contaminated blood. Most important, human hybridoma cell lines are very unstable, which usually blocks the road to monoclonal human antibodies.

Human antibodies, however, are especially favored over those from other animals when used *in vivo* for diagnosis or therapy. They could save a patient from pathogens or poisons and they might help in the fight against cancer due to their specificity. Their main advantage is their human origin, which prevents the patient from launching an immune response against the antibody, which not only neutralizes e.g. a mouse monoclonal antibody but sometimes even endangers the patient (see Section 2.4.2). Therefore, the production of human antibodies by means of gene technology has allowed for *in vivo* diagnostic and therapeutic strategies that cannot be conducted with common methods.

1.2.6.3 Antibodies Fused To Other Proteins Gain Completely New Properties

Even a "normal" antibody is a *bifunctional* molecule. While the variable moiety binds to its specific antigen, the constant moiety determines what happens to the marked molecule, with other parts of the immune system called in.

Similarly, the antigen-binding site can be genetically fused with a nearly unlimited variety of other proteins. Thus, the antibody-binding portions can be grafted with biochemical functions that would not be found in such a combination in nature. For example, an enzyme can be specifically targeted to a tumor cell with the aid of an antibody fragment; this bifunctional antibody (see Section 3.3) is a potential therapeutic tool against cancer.

An especially interesting fusion links two different antigen-binding sites into one, *bispecific antibody* (see Section 3.2). One antibody fragment could bind, for example, to a tumor cell and the other could then activate the immune system and, as such, perhaps fulfill the long-cherished dream of cancer researchers for a therapy that provides the body with an immunological defense against cancer.

Consideration of the three-dimensional structure of the variable regions of immunoglobulins indicates that the structural prerequisites for such constructs exist (see Fig. 1.2) The carboxy termini of the individual regions each lie on the side of the molecule opposite to that of the antigen-binding site. This permits larger polypeptides to be genetically conjugated to the carboxy termini, without causing any steric hindrance to antigen binding. Genetic conjugates can be produced as continuous fusion proteins, made up from many different components, by connecting the variable chains of an antibody with a peptide linker.

These genetic fusions produced through recombination have advantages over the common methods for coupling proteins because the coupling locus and the stoichiometry of both partners are precisely defined. The ever-present risk of destruction of the antigen-binding site, during chemical covalent modification with a coupling agent, is hereby eliminated. Additionally, there is no need to remove unwanted by-products of a chemical reaction. With genetic fusion, multiple coupling of a whole range of components from different proteins is possible, which cannot be constructed at all using common methods.

Therefore, recombinant antibodies have expanded the horizon to a wide spectrum of different applications of antigen-binding proteins. However, recombinant technology will never entirely replace the established methods of antibody production, but rather merge with them.

References

Janeway CA, Travers P (1997) Immunologie. Spektrum Akademischer Verlag, Heidelberg.

Kabat EA, Wu TT, Reid-Miller M, Perry HM, Gottesman KS (1987) Sequences of Proteins of Immunological Interest, US Dept. of Health and Human Services, US Government Printing Office, Washington, DC.

Köhler G, Milstein C (1975) Continuous cultures of fused cells secreting antibody of predefined specificity. *Nature* **256**:495–497.

Liddell E, Weeks I (1996) Antikörpertechniken. Spektrum Akademischer Verlag, Heidelberg.

Chapter 2
Building Recombinant Antibody Fragments

2.1 Introduction

2.1.1 BACTERIA CAN PRODUCE RECOMBINANT ANTIBODY FRAGMENTS

It took a long time before the first functionally competent antibody fragment could be produced in *E. coli*. This was probably due to the fact that antibodies are truly complex molecules, formed from two chains. In eukaryotic cells, the chains are folded correctly with the aid of antibody-specific helper proteins, or *chaperones* (Bornemann et al., 1995; Kirkpatrick et al., 1995). Moreover, both chains are stabilized through internal disulfide bonds, which require an oxidative biochemical environment for their formation. The real breakthrough in solving this problem came with the fusion of the antibody gene to a bacterial *signal sequence*, which causes the secretion of the antibody fragment into the *periplasmic* space (Skerra and Plückthun, 1988; Better et al., 1998). The periplasmic space is located between the two cell membranes of the bacterium and, in contrast to the cytoplasm, contains a biochemical environment in which the antibodies can be folded correctly. Only here can the disulfide bridges within the antibody regions be properly formed. Additionally, the bacterial chaperones of this compartment are better suited to their task than those of the cytoplasm (see also Section 4.2.1.1)

2.1.2 THE HUMORAL IMMUNE SYSTEM CAN BE IMITATED IN BACTERIA

After this initial breakthrough, the way was free to emulate the decisive steps of antibody formation of the mammalian immune system in bacteria. These are based essentially on three principles (Fig. 2.1):
1. Availability of a large number of antibody genes
2. Effective selection of the correct gene from this pool
3. Improvement in the affinity and specificity of a selected antibody fragment

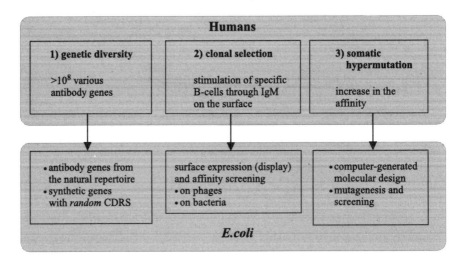

Fig. 2.1. The three fundamental principles of the human antibody immune response can be imitated in *E. coli*.

The key to producing recombinant antibodies lies in the transferral of these principles into experimentally manageable systems. Only then can antibody fragments be altered with comparative ease and be equipped with new properties. This is especially simple to achieve in *E. coli*, the showcase of modern molecular biology (Fuchs et al., 1992; Winter et al., 1994; de Kruif et al., 1996; Hayden et al., 1997). The following three sections describe accordingly how this "carry over of the immune response into the test tube" was successfully achieved.

2.1.2.1 Antibody variety in *E. coli*

As described in the introduction, the wide range of human antibody genes arises from the random combination of gene fragments. Each B-lymphocyte accordingly acquires its own unique antibody gene. The information for this enormous repertoire of genes is then stored in the body as a pool of B-lymphocytes. As a result, it is estimated that man has more than 10^8 different antibody genes at his disposal.

This gene pool can be accessed with the help of the *polymerase chain reaction* (PCR). Two oligonucleotide primers that complement the termini of the desired antibody gene can be used to amplify the portion of the DNA that lies in between. Using this method, not only can individual genes be amplified, but also entire gene families, such as the complete antibody gene family. The information for this set of genes is found in the cDNA obtained from B-lymphocyte mRNA (Fig. 2.2). If, at the same time, the oligonucleotide primers introduce restriction sites into the antibody gene, the antibody genes can be incorporated into *E. coli* expression vectors. Thus, the information for a nearly limitless number of antibody genes has been transferred to the test tube. A few micrograms of plasmid DNA contain around 10^{11} plasmids that, because of the new combinations of the heavy and light chains, hardly ever code for

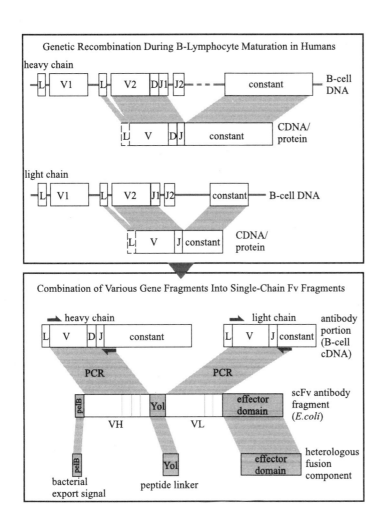

Fig. 2.2. The source of the antibody genes. **(Top)** During the natural development of the B-lymphocyte repertoire in the body, each B-lymphocyte develops the gene for its specific antibody by recombination of V, J, and D sequences. The information for the complete set of antibody genes is found in a mixture of B-lymphocytes—more precisely, in their mRNA. **(Bottom)** The information can be obtained from here with the help of the polymerase chain reaction (PCR). The VH and the VL genes of the antibodies are amplified with two oligonucleotide primers each (represented with gray half-arrows) that hybridize to both ends of the desired gene fragment. The resulting gene fragments are combined with DNA fragments from other organisms and assembled into scFv genes. Thus, the properties of the desired recombinant protein can be adapted for an optimized production in *E. coli*. In the example illustrated here, the two antibody chains of a scFv fragment are linked into a single protein by a peptide of 15–18 amino acids. A bacterial signal sequence (pel B) is fused to the N-terminus of the protein that causes secretion through the inner membrane of the *E. coli* cell. The resulting gene for an scFv fragment can be lengthened by nearly any other gene fragment, through which it gains additional biochemical properties.

the same antibody fragments. The complexity of the bacterial antibody library now only depends on the highest possible efficiency method of transformation. The best antibody libraries achieve a complexity of about 10^{10} different antibody genes. The construction of such libraries is comprehensively discussed in Section 2.2.

2.1.2.2 The Surface Expression of Antibodies Allows for a Clonal Selection

The second principle was more difficult to realize in bacteria: the selection of the desired antibody from the antibody pool, that is, a clonal selection. Initially, attempts were made to achieve a large quantity of antibody-producing clones on agar plates. This method, however, rarely enabled a selection from 10^6 or more clones (Huse et al., 1989). Additionally, this method produces antibody fragments that are membrane-bound and, therefore, often denatured. An improved selection method was necessary to facilitate access to an antibody gene repertoire that somewhat resembled that of humans.

Again, the example set by nature was of help. A human B-lymphocyte first presents its antibodies membrane-bound on the surface (Fig. 2.3). On contact with the specific antigen, the B-lymphocyte is activated and begins to multiply. This proliferation of a specific cell out of the B-lymphocyte pool is called *clonal selection* because it results in a large number of descendants from a single cell, that is, a clone. The solution also lay in the physical connection of the antibody with the gene that codes for it. In the form of a B-lymphocyte, the antibody carries its own piggyback gene. Antigen binding then allows for a selective proliferation of this particle. Today, there are a large number of methods that mimic these features. Antibody fragments were fused with surface proteins from bacteria, retroviruses or baculoviruses. In the most frequently used method, especially small particles are generated where the antibody fragments are displayed on the surface of a filamentous bacteriophage. Two examples are illustrated in Figure 2.3 and the detailed description of various methods follows in Section 2.3.

2.1.2.3 Somatic Hypermutation in Bacteria

The third principle of the humoral immune response can also be transferred into bacteria with the aid of an efficient selection system. An improved affinity and specificity of antigen binding is achieved in our immune system through *somatic hypermutation*. Here, random mutations are introduced into the antibody genes of already preselected B-lymphocytes, that present antigen-specific antibodies on their surface. Thereafter the cells, whose mutated antibodies bind antigen better, are selectively multiplied. The efficient selection system described above enables this principle to be transferred into bacteria. Again, a large number of mutations are introduced into the antibody sequences later to select the better antigen-binder, this time in *E. coli*. In this way, more than a hundredfold improvement of the binding constant of an antibody fragment could be achieved. More details are discussed in Section 2.4.

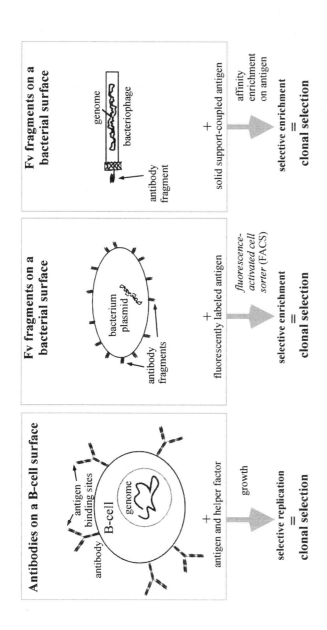

Fig. 2.3. Clonal selection in the immune system and in bacteria. **(Left)** The clonal selection of a B-lymphocyte. Proliferation of the B-lymphocyte is triggered by its contact with antigen. This contact is mediated by an antigen-specific antibody presented by 'its' B-lymphocyte. Thus, together with the antibody the gene encoding it is amplified. Two systems are illustrated in the middle and on the right that help to imitate this process in *E. coli*. **(Middle)** When an antibody is presented on the surface of a bacterium, its gene (together with the bacterium) can be selected with the help of a fluorescently labeled antigen and a fluorescence-activated cell sorter (FACS). **(Right)** When an antibody fragment is anchored on the surface of a phage particle, the whole particle can thus be bound to antigen. The antibody gene is thereby coenriched.

2.2 Sources of Antibody Genes

2.2.1 COMBINATORIAL ASSEMBLY OF ANTIBODY GENES

Our germline genome provides for the building-blocks finally to be assembled into functional antibody genes. Apart from the Fc-regions, the biggest piece of antibody gene is coded for by the V regions of the heavy and light chains. The VH *locus* comprises 51 functional genes that are distributed over 1,100 kb of the genome, with a similar number of pseudogenes (Cook and Tomlinson, 1995). The 52 human V lambda genes are distributed over 800 kb (Frippiat et al., 1995), and for the kappa chains, 40 functional genes are available (Tomlinson et al., 1995). These V genes are combined with further gene segments, the J and D genes. In order to obtain a functional antibody gene, one of these V genes is randomly ligated to one of the J genes, with one additional D gene spliced in between VH and JH gene segments.

The result of this process is a variety of B-lymphocytes, each coding for a different antibody, due to an individual combination of the different gene segments. In addition, mutations and extensions are generated, especially, in the CDR3 of the heavy chain. Thus, our immune system generates more than 100 million different antibodies with the potential to recognize nearly every antigen.

The above-mentioned genomic V genes correspond to only a portion of the V region of recombinant antibody fragments, while the term *variable region* or *variable domain* is reserved for the whole Fv portion of the heavy or light chains. In contrast to the V genes, the V region also comprises the CDR3 and the *framework-4* regions coded for by J genes (or D and J genes), on the genome. Opinions differ about the length of the variable domain. The most commonly used convention places the end of the V regions at amino acid 113 for the VH region and 109 for the VL region (Kabat et al., 1987).

2.2.2 COMPLEXITY OF ANTIBODY GENE LIBRARIES

As already mentioned in the introduction, the whole set of antibody genes can be amplified with the help of PCR (see Mullis et al., 1992; Newton and Graham, 1994). This results into an antibody gene library in the test tube, from which individual antibodies can be isolated by clonal selection. Theoretically, it is sufficient to produce an antibody gene library only once. This library should approximate the complexity of the human immune repertoire in which nearly every potential antibody is represented. In practice, however, this has proved difficult. First, the transformation efficiency is limited (this determines the complexity of the antibody gene library), and second, the capability of the selection system is pushed to its limits. Added to this, the production and cultivation of very large libraries require enormous effort. According to the goal, libraries of different complexities are produced, ranging from just a few up to 10^{10} different sequences (Fig. 2.4).

Complexity of the
Antibody repertoire

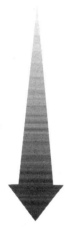

1. PCR with cDNA from defined cell lines (myeloma, hybridoma)

2. PCR with cDNA from seropositive donor (IgG library of activated B-cells)

3. PCR with cDNA from a nonimmunized donor = native repertoire (IgM library of nonactivated B-cells)

4. PCR from genomic DNA (the whole of the variable regions)

5. *random* oligonucleotides for hypervariable regions

Fig. 2.4.   Antibody gene libraries of different complexities.

For some applications a pre-existing hybridome can deliver the antibody genes desired. If this source is not available, an antibody gene library must be produced, from which the desired antibody fragment can be selected. Often for this purpose, the best source of antibody genes are the B-lymphocytes from the blood of an immunized donor. This preselects for antigen-specific antibody genes and hence library sizes of a million independent clones usually suffice to achieve the desired recombinant antibody fragment. Only when an immunization is not possible is it necessary to start with "universal" antibody gene libraries. However, very complex libraries with a minimum of 10^8 independent clones are needed in order to obtain recombinant antibody fragments of sufficient affinity. The cost of production and propagation rises accordingly. The best currently available libraries comprise more than 10^{10} independent clones, and therefore, probably the majority of antibody genes coded for by the human immune system (Nissim et al., 1994). Theoretically, the oligonucleotide synthesis of random sequences should enable an even greater complexity, because nature provides only a limited set of varying sequences for each hypervariable region. The astronomical complexity that is theoretically possible is, however, no longer practical.

An overview of the commonly used methods of producing libraries is given in Figure 2.5. Of course, mixed forms of the respective libraries can also be produced, such as donor libraries, in which a hypervariable region is additionally randomized, that is, supplemented with synthetic, random sequences. Some of the "universal" libraries in use are, indeed, such mixed forms. Here the phage particles from very differently constructed libraries are combined to form a common library of greater complexity. The different types of libraries, their production and uses, are discussed in detail in the following section.

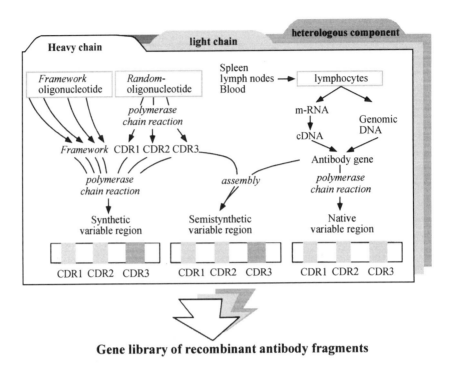

Gene library of recombinant antibody fragments

Fig. 2.5.   Getting the genes of the variable regions into antibody libraries.

2.2.3 WHAT IS THE REAL COMPLEXITY OF ANTIBODY GENE LIBRARIES?

Once PCR, restriction digestion, ligation, and transformation have been accomplished in the construction of a library, the question arises whether any of the calculated complexity of the library is lost during these procedures. The first step is, of course, to determine the number of independent clones present after the transformation of *E. coli*. Dilutions of the library are plated out onto agar and the number of colonies yields a measure of the library complexity. The determination of the proportion of productive clones is also relatively easy. A few hundred bacterial clones are lifted onto nitrocellulose filters (plate screen or *colony lift assay*) and then the expression of antibody genes is detected with an antibody-specific reagent (Dübel et al., 1995; Song et al., 1997). If the library comprises more than a few thousand independent clones, obtaining direct evidence about the actual complexity is unfortunately no longer possible. The reason for this lies in the laws of statistics. If a sample is to be used to draw conclusions about the overall complexity, this sample must represent at least 1% of the total. In an average library of 10^8 independent clones, at least 1 million clones would have to be tested.

In order to get an indication about the quality of the library, a large number of randomly isolated clones can be digested with the help of the restriction enzyme BstNI (Marks et al., 1991a). This enzyme distinguishes itself in that the distribution of its recognition sequences in antibody DNA is highly polymorphic. Different sequences can be identified when differing restriction patterns are observed. However, in no way does an identical pattern prove the identity of the sequences.

More informative, but comparatively more laborious, is the sequencing of some 100 clones from the antibody library. This tests if the obtained sequences are to be found in the same statistical distribution as in the parent antibody gene library (Welschof et al., 1995). In the end, the only way to gain an indication of the real complexity is by the successful isolation of antibodies with different antigens. A rule of thumb is that the larger libraries allow the isolation of higher affinity antibodies.

In terms of evolution, *E. coli* bacteria have diverged from either man or mouse for hundreds of millions of years. Therefore, expression of human antibody genes in these bacteria brings about a further, hard-to-estimate reduction in the actual complexity:

1. A few human DNA sequences are not replicated by *E. coli* or they retard growth. Out of a mixture of different sequences, such sequences are already removed during cloning because the bacteria that contain them either cannot survive, or remove the sequences by deletion.
2. Most amino acids are coded for by several nucleotide triplets because the genetic code is degenerate. The triplets preferred by *E. coli* (reflected in the sets of corresponding tRNAs) are therefore different from those preferred by human cells (Grosjean and Fiers, 1982). This means that some human antibody genes are only poorly read in *E. coli*, and thus occur less often in the library produced for the selection process.
3. The apparatus for producing, translocating, and folding proteins is clearly different in *E. coli* compared to mammals, and this causes a structural incompatibility. Different antibodies fold with very different efficiencies in *E. coli*. Even the exchange of a single amino acid can have a dramatic effect on the yield of soluble fragments (Chapter 4). As a result, a strong selective pressure affects the production of soluble antibody fragments, particularly in the expression of antibody genes.
4. The recombinant antibody fragments that are produced must not react with the host. Thus, isolating antibodies against *E. coli* surface proteins from an *E. coli*/phage library is very difficult.

Consequently, the number of independent clones never suggests the true number of available recombinant antibody fragments. By the same token, the actual complexity cannot be determined. The complexity figures that are given in the literature are to be understood more as a convention that reflects the cost of producing the library.

2.2.4 CLONING ANTIBODY GENES FROM HYBRIDOMA CELL LINES

To obtain scFv fragments from hybridoma cell lines, the two gene fragments for the light chains must first be obtained. Most practically this is done by PCR using antibody-specific oligonucleotide primers (Huse et al., 1989; Orlandi et al., 1989; Songsivilai et al., 1990; Dübel et al., 1994). The direct cloning of antibody genes from hybridoma cell lines was the first attempt at producing recombinant antibody fragments. It was already used in the production of new fusion proteins before the development of more effective, *in vitro* selection procedures, such as phage display. To cite an example, a plasminogen activator could bind fibrin more effectively when fused to the heavy chain of a recombinant antibody (Schnee et al., 1987).

In contrast to most other PCR applications, the reaction conditions for the PCR amplification of antibody genes must be optimized for *low* specificity. The reason for this is that the antibody gene to be amplified usually does not perfectly match the oligonucleotide primer. This, again, lies in the diversity of rearranged antibody genes. For the V regions of the antibody alone, the mouse genome contains more than 100 different sequences that still could be additionally, somatically mutated. Extensive oligonucleotide primer sets can be constructed for the amplification (e.g., Orlandi et al., 1989; Marks et al., 1991a; Campbell et al., 1992; Ørum et al., 1993), in which each member matches to a different partner within the various antibody sequences. This approach makes sense in the production of highly complex antibody gene libraries, from which antibodies against various antigens are to be obtained at a later date (see below). To this end, amplifying the whole repertoire of various sequences in equimolar quantities is worthwhile because, at the outset, it is not known which of the chains possess the desired specificity. From a financial viewpoint, however, when cloning from hybridomas, starting with a small number of oligonucleotide primers is preferable. Amplifying all the sequences should nevertheless still be possible. Such an oligonucleotide primer set, used to amplify mouse and rat Fv DNA (from Dübel et al., 1994), is presented in Table 2.1.

In the particular case shown in Table 2.1 the 3' oligonucleotide primers hybridize to the conserved portion of the constant chain directly adjacent to the framework 4 region of the variable region. As such, only a single primer is required for each 3' end. The 5' oligonucleotide primers are relatively long, and mixtures of several nucleotides (wobbles) are incorporated at certain positions. This design ensures that at least one from each set of three varying mixtures should hybridize to all known mouse sequences. The oligonucleotide primers shown were successfully used in the amplification of antibody genes from more

Table 2.1 **Oligonucleotides for the amplication of DNA from the variable regions of mouse and rat immunoglobulins**

Region of Hybridization	Primer No.	Sequence (5'–3')
Variable region of the light chain	6	GGTGATATCGTGAT(A/G)AC(C/A)CA(G/A)GATGAACTCTC
	7	GGTGATATC(A/T)TG(A/C)TGACCCAA(A/T)CTCCACTCTC
	8	GGTGATATCGT(G/T)CTCAC(C/T)CA(A/G)TCTCCAGCAAT
κ constant region	5	GGGAAGATGGATCCAGTTGGTGCAGCATCAGC
Variable region of the heavy chain	3	GAGGTGAAGCTGCAGGAGTCAGGACCTAGCCTGGTG
	3b	AGGT(C/G)(A/C)AACTGCAG(C/G)AGTC(A/T)GG
	3c	AGGT(C/G)(A/C)AGCTGCAG(C/G)AGTC(A/T)GG
γ constant region	4	CCAGGGGCCAGTGGATAGACAAGCTTGGGTGTCGTTTT

than 30 different mouse and rat hybridomas (Dübel et al., 1994), with a comprehensive laboratory protocol for the cloning of scFv fragments from hybridomas published in Breitling and Dübel (1997).

2.2.4.1 Hybridoma Cell Lines Used to Produce Monoclonal Antibodies Are Genetically Heterogeneous

In the amplification of antibody genes from hybridoma cell lines, different antibody sequences are continually being found (Fuchs et al., 1997) even though hybridoma cell lines are described as monoclonal. The term monoclonal stems historically from the detection of an antibody of desired specificity in cell culture medium. The myeloma fusion partner is optimized to express the least possible amount of its own, unwanted, antibody genes. Despite this, these unwanted chains (or other, weakly expressed pseudogenes), can be amplified through PCR (H. Zhang, unpublished results). This also applies for mutations that accumulate in the hybridomal antibody genes during an extended cultivation of the hybridoma. It is therefore advisable to start with hybridoma cultures that are freshly subcloned and tested, when obtaining hybridomal, antibody cDNA. A further source of unwanted mutations is added by the use of degenerate PCR primers. With the low-stringency-conditions used, these primers do not need a perfect match in order to hybridize. Therefore, a quick test on the function of the scFv fragments is essential. With soluble antigen at hand, phage display vectors are surely the method of choice (discussed in Section 2.3 and following sections). Although difficult, this also works as well with membrane-bound antigens on cell surfaces (Marks et al., 1993; Dziegiel et al., 1995; de Kruif et al., 1995b).

Without an easy test system at hand, the genetic heterogeneity must be analyzed by sequencing at least 10 clones per region. If different sequences appear, all possible combinations of VH and VL should be produced separately and functionally tested.

2.2.4.2 Oligonucleotide Primers for the Generation of Antibody Gene Libraries

The selection methods described in detail in Section 2.3, enable a single, recombinant antibody fragment to be picked out from millions, provided that the fragment of desired specificity is actually present, somewhere within the library. Because of this, the complexity of expression libraries is crucial for success. In contrast to the cloning of antibodies from hybridoma cells, the production of a good antibody gene library must fulfil a further condition; as many existing antibody genes as possible should be amplified by PCR in *equimolar* quantities. Otherwise, precisely the V-region of choice could be overwhelmed by the other sequences and later, may be lost. A primer set has been developed by Welschof and colleagues (1995), for example, which fulfils this criterion for human antibody sequences. The strategy employed is illustrated in Figure 2.6. A total of 100 randomly selected clones were amplified in this way and sequenced. This showed that libraries produced with this

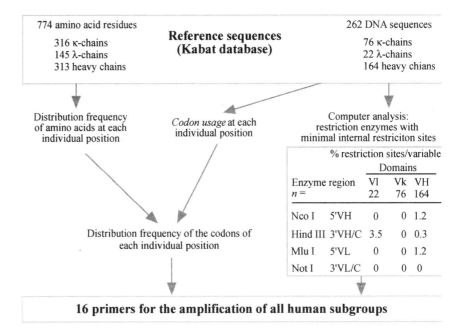

Fig. 2.6. Oligonucleotide primer design strategies for the amplification of antibody cDNA.

method contain the natural distribution of subclasses and that functional recombinant antibody fragments against many different antigens can be extracted (Welschof et al., 1997a) (M. Little, personal communication). A detailed protocol for the production of a human scFv library can be found in Welschof et al., (1997b).

Other primer sets of marginally differing design have also been used successfully to amplify human antibody DNA (Orlandi et al., 1989; Marks et al., 1991a; Campbell et al., 1992). Meanwhile, all genomic sequences of human antibody V regions are known, so that amplifying any one chain should be possible, at least from human DNA. Similarly abundant, oligonucleotide primers are also available for the mouse (Ørum et al., 1993).

Particularly simple primer sets can be constructed for the amplification of DNA from rabbit antibody V regions. In these animals, gene conversion generates the diversity of antibody sequences. Therefore, the conserved ends of the Fv regions can be used to amplify the whole set of antibody genes indiscriminately (Ridder et al., 1995).

To save on work, some groups use an *overlap* or *assembly* PCR. First, the two V regions are amplified in two independent PCR reactions. Provided the oligonucleotide primer code for the peptide linker in between the V regions and overlap with each other, the two V regions can be assembled into a single piece of DNA in a third round of PCR (Fig. 2.7). The disadvantage of this method lies in the susceptibility for PCR artifacts. Thus, an increased number of clones with shortened linkers are found in libraries produced by this method (J. D. Marks, personal communication).

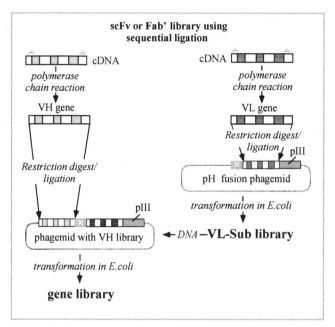

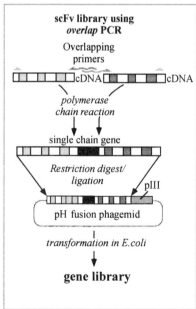

Fig. 2.7. Getting the antibody diversity into the test tube. Various PCR methods are used in order to amplify the information stored in the mRNA of B-lymphocytes. Half-arrows: oligonucteotide primers for PCR; all-white boxes: variable region of the heavy chain; black and white boxes: variable region of the light chain; X: linker peptide (in scFv libraries) or ribosomal binding site and signal peptide (in Fv or Fab' libraries).

2.2.4.3 The Combinatorial Assembly of the Variable Heavy and Light Regions Increases the Complexity of an Antibody Gene Library

In the techniques described above, a novel combination of the two V regions occurs *in vitro*. DNA from a particular VH region is randomly combined with all VL region DNA fragments. Therefore, the theoretical complexity of the antibody gene library multiplies through the multiplication of the complexities of the VH and VL component libraries. This can be a desired result when producing a "universal" library. It can be disadvantageous, however, when the aim is to select for a particular, existing antibody from the blood of an immunized donor, because the desired pairing of the variable domains is diluted among the "wrong" or, more appropriately, "not original" pairings.

These new combinations can be limited by *in cell* PCR. This is a method where the genes for the variable domains are amplified and combined *in situ*, which is still in the antibody-producing cells (Embleton et al., 1992). Thereby the natural combination of heavy and light chains is conserved. A library based on this technique would represent the antibodies originally produced by the donor. This is of special interest, if recombinant antibody fragments are desired that descend from such an original antibody (e.g. an antibody elicited by immunization). However, the proficiency of this approach in the construction of an antibody gene library must still be proven.

2.2.5 GENE LIBRARIES FROM IMMUNIZED DONORS

When the desired antibody is detectable in the serum of the donor, a rough estimate assumes that one in every thousand plasma cells produces this antibody. Plasma cells harbor many copies of the corresponding mRNA, typically of the IgG Subgroup. Therefore, the method of choice employs IgG-specific oligonucleotide primers for the isolation and amplification of the cDNA for the heavy chain. Due to the random combination of VH and VL, the original combination of the desired antibody can be expected in a thousand times a thousand clones. Libraries of 10^6 independent clones are therefore usually sufficient for immunized donors.

2.2.5.1 Antibody Gene Libraries derived from Immunized humans

Producing human monoclonal antibodies with conventional hybridoma technology is very difficult. Recombinant antibodies offer a way out of this dilemma by the use of human antibody gene libraries. A targeted immunization of humans is only possible in rare cases, yet a number of interesting antibodies can still be obtained. An especially interesting source of antibody genes are people who have already developed an appropriate immune response resulting from an illness. Usually only 10 ml of blood is necessary from which a patient library can be made. As an example, a number of partly neutralizing antivirus antibodies have already been isolated (Zebedee et al., 1992; Williamson et al., 1993). A second important area of use is the research into autoimmune diseases. Various potential autoantibodies could be identified with the help of patient libraries, for example, against thyroidperioxidase (Portolano et al., 1993), against U1 RNA, a marker in patients with systemic lupus erythematosus (Powers et al., 1995), or a potential immune-regulating anti-(Fab)$_2$ - antibody (Welschof et al., 1997a). Patient libraries therefore offer a new way to access the antibodies that are otherwise difficult to obtain. Often, they also open avenues to new types of therapies. They are now the method of choice to obtain human antibody fragments.

An interesting variation in the production of human antibodies is offered by the immunization of an SCID mouse (severe combined immune deficiency). These mice lack their own specific immune system and can be populated with human peripheral lymphocytes. When these human lymphocytes comprise memory B-lymphocytes, it is possible to stimulate them into a second, strong, immune response with antigen. Specific human antibody fragments then can be isolated from an antibody library that is produced as described above (Duchosal et al., 1992).

2.2.5.2 Antibody Gene Libraries Derived From Immunized Mice

Libraries that are based on antibody genes from immunized mice have also proved successful (e.g., Ørum et al., 1993). Additionally, mice can be immunized with any antigen that is not desirable for use in man, for example, polysaccharide epitopes from plants (Williams et al., 1996). Cell type-specific antibodies can also be obtained by this method. In the cited example, after immunization with a particular type of neuron, antibody fragments against its surface proteins can be obtained (Merz et al., 1995).

A particularly interesting example is that of a recombinant antibody that recognizes an MHC molecule, only when it is laden with a specific peptide (Andersen et al., 1996). The antibody obviously recognizes the peptide–MHC complex in a way similar to the T-cell receptor (Stryhn et al., 1996). In other words, this recombinant antibody recognizes specific peptides that stem from the inside of the cell. The amino acids of the antibody that are responsible for the specific peptide binding might be successfully identified. If these are replaced with random amino acids, an antibody library would result from which other peptide-specific antibodies could be isolated. Perhaps one day, these could be used to eliminate virus-infected cells.

The use of mice offers the additional advantage that two different methods for producing monoclonal antibodies can be used in parallel. Next to the recombinant method, half the spleen can be used for the classical hybridoma production. Due to the different selection systems, the two methods could lead to different antibodies, as was observed in the case of antibodies generated with both methods against IL-5 (Ames et al., 1995).

2.2.5.3 Antibody Gene Libraries From Other Donor Animals (Rabbit, Chicken)

Other types of animals have also been used successfully in the production of antibody gene libraries. Emphasis is placed especially on the rabbit, which for years has been used in numerous laboratories as an excellent provider of antibodies (Ridder et al., 1995; Lang et al., 1996). Chickens have increasingly been used for the production of antisera for some time because of the ability to extract antibodies in a bloodless fashion from eggs. Chickens were already used successfully for the production of recombinant antibody fragments from libraries (Davies et al., 1995; Yamanaka et al., 1996). An ample experimental infrastructure (e.g., purification and detection agents) already exists for antibodies from both species, because of their widespread use in the production of antibodies by conventional methods (see Chapter 4).

2.2.6 UNIVERSAL ANTIBODY GENE LIBRARIES FROM NONIMMUNIZED DONORS

IgM-specific oligonucleotide primers enable access to the naive, antibody repertoire of man. Such primers usually amplify only the heavy-chain DNA from B-lymphocytes that have not yet been clonally stimulated with antigen. B-lymphocytes such as these produce a membrane-bound form of IgM (mIgM) and represent the repertoire that is available to the naive immune system of man in an antibody response. After stimulating with antigen, the genes are rearranged resulting in the class switch, which usually leads to the expression of IgGs. In contrast to the activated B-lymphocytes mostly concentrated in lymphatic organs, the IgM-producing types of B cells also circulate in the peripheral bloodstream of humans, from which the genes can be extracted very easily. If the IgM specific primers are exchanged for PCR-primers that hybridize in the V region (more precisely, in framework 4), the VH genes that have already performed an isotope switch and clonal amplification are amplified as well. Such libraries yield antibody fragments against all important types of antigen (proteins, cell surface markers, peptides, haptens, such as steroids, and sugar complexes) (Marks et al., 1991b; 1993; Griffiths et al., 1993; Hughes-Jones et al., 1994; reviewed in Lerner et al., 1992). However, the effort of making and maintaining such a universal library is only worthwhile when a large number of different antibodies need to be produced.

2.2.6.1 Universal Antibody Gene Libraries From Mouse B-Lymphocytes

The main impetus for the generation of universal antibody gene libraries was the search for human antibodies, especially those eliminated during the development of an immune response, or whose antigens rendered an immunization impossible. Despite the great effort necessary, attempts were also made to make use of these advantages in the favored animal of the immunologists: the mouse. The antibodies obtained in this way did not, however, achieve the affinity of the recombinant antibody fragments obtained from immunized mice (Gram et al., 1992).

2.2.7 GENOMIC ANTIBODY GENE LIBRARIES

Cloning of the total, genomic, V gene repertoire of man opened a new source for the construction of "universal" antibody gene libraries. In this approach the individual gene fragments of the V region are not obtained as rearranged antibody genes from B-cell DNA, but similar to the rearrangement procedure, they are newly put together *in vitro*. In the mean time, recombinant antibody fragments, against a large number of different antigens, have been isolated from such a library (Nissim et al., 1994).

A completely different type of genomic library is are illustrated in mice, whose own immunoglobulin gene locus was replaced with portions of the human immunoglobulin gene locus. The human antibody genes rearrange, perform the *class switch* and are somatically hypermutated. These transgenic mice then produce human antibodies in mouse cells, which, in contrast to human hybridoma cells, lead to stable mouse hybridomas (Jakobovits, 1995; Lonberg and Huszar, 1995). Unfortunately, these mice are currently only accessible for commercial applications.

2.2.8 HYBRID AND SEMISYNTHETIC ANTIBODY GENE LIBRARIES

The methods described in the previous sections can also be combined. A library from the VH genes of peripheral blood lymphocytes from an alloimmunized donor was combined with the VL gene regions from a nonimmunized donor. From this, library antibodies specific for polymorphic thrombocyte glycoproteins were selected that could not be obtained with conventional hybridoma technology (Griffin and Ouwehand, 1995).

Sequence comparisons show that the CDR3 of the heavy chain is the most variable portion of the antibody sequence. The extraordinary role of these CDRs in antibody binding has been confirmed by structural data. Our immune system generates a large portion of the variability in the area of the CDR3 by random synthesis. A mere sidestep from this was to mutate these and/or further CDRs in the antibody gene library with random sequences, to improve the scope of the library. Since then, a large number of antibodies have been successfully isolated from such *semisynthetic genomic libraries* (Barbas et al., 1992; Akamatsu et al., 1993; de Kruif et al., 1995a; de Wildt et al., 1996; Dinh et al., 1996).

2.2.9 SYNTHETIC ANTIBODY GENE LIBRARIES WITH RANDOM SEQUENCES IN THE CDRs

Among the antibodies generated through the random combination of its building blocks are a few antibodies directed against epitopes of body itself. Such antibodies can lead to autoimmune diseases. Normally, the B-lymphocytes encoding these antibodies are suppressed during the development of the immune system. A few of these deleted specificities, however, are of interest in tumor therapy, for example, antigens from embryonic or dedifferentiated human cells. This limitation does not exist in synthetically produced gene libraries in *E. coli*. Therefore, the completely synthetic production of antibody genes, with random sequences in all the CDRs, has been attempted many times over (Hayashi et al., 1994; Braunagel, 1995; Soderlind et al., 1995). It appeared that the synthesis of multiple, randomized sequences by *overlap* PCR can be successfully used in the synthesis of such antibody gene libraries. However, analysis of these libraries shows a high error rate through mutations, synthesis errors and PCR artifacts. Additionally, these antibody gene libraries do not represent truly random sequences, because the complexity must be restricted to avoid stop codons occurring in the random regions. In a random sequence $(NNN)_n$, three stop codons in 64 triplets are expected. This rate would lead to hardly any sequences being fully read, in antibodies with several randomized CDRs. It is more profitable to use $(NNK)_n$, where K = G or T. This yields a stop codon in one of 32 codons, and all the amino acids are still represented. Today, $(NNB)_n$ is common, where B = G or T or C. This yields a stop codon in one of 48 codons, and here too, all amino acids are represented. All these sequences, however, code for the different amino acids at different frequencies. As such, the amino acids arginine and serine in the triplet $(NNB)_n$ are represented four times more frequently than methionine or tryptophan. A good overview of synthetic gene libraries is given by Arkin and Youvan (1992).

If all the CDRs of a Fv fragment are to be randomized, avoiding stop codons in full is desirable. This is possible with $(VNN)_n$ for example, where V = A, G, or C. Here, however, it must be accepted that a few amino acids will not be coded for at all (in our example, 4 of the possible 20), and also that the distribution of the remaining ones does not correspond to their natural occurrence. The use of oligonucleotide mixtures, with variable portions at particular position, (e.g., 32% A, 32% C, 32% G, and 4% T instead of V for the above example), also permits a limited number of the four, missing amino acids, although at the price of a few stop codons. If all the CDRs are simultaneously fully randomized, the proportion of functional antibodies in such libraries will be only very small, because of the extremely high number of possible structures. Therefore, a reduction in the randomization of the CDRs is certainly preferred. It should be limited to the relatively few amino acids that come into contact with the antigen (see Section 4.1.1).

Recently, a solution to the problems described above has arisen. Instead of mononucleotide building blocks, oligonucleotides are assembled from trinucleotide elements (Sondek and Shortle, 1992; Virnekas et al., 1994; Lyttle et al., 1995). Every protein sequence can be produced with 20 different trinucleotides, because each trinucleotide codes exactly for one amino acid. This completely avoids stop codons. Additionally, this method allows for the insertion of mixtures of trinucleotides. Preferred amino acids have been found in many sites of the CDRs, whose role can often additionally be explained by their structure. To account for this, with the help of trinucleotide synthesis, only combinations of amino acids with small side chains, or only hydrophobic, or any favored choice can be inserted. Thus, the number of sequences, which should allow for natural folding, can be drastically increased.

2.2.10 IN VIVO RECOMBINATION SYSTEMS ENABLE "SUPERLIBRARIES"

The antigen-binding site of the antibody is composed of the variable domains of the heavy and light chains, with the random combination of these two chains largely conributing to the huge variety of antibody genes. This random combination also occurs in the test tube by the ligation of the recombinant antibody into a plasmid vector. On this level, an almost unbelievable range of different antibodies exists, as almost every plasmid should be able to code for a unique antibody. The bottleneck in the construction of highly complex libraries lies in the next step, that is, the transformation of the plasmid DNA into competent bacteria. Using the best available method, electroporation, antibody libraries with more than 10^7 independent clones can be achieved routinely. This also means that constructing combinatorial libraries with this level of complexity is possible, hence a library with some 10^7 different heavy chains and a second with some 10^7 different light chains. The great efficiency with which the filamentous phage infects its host bacteria can then be exploited to combine the millionfold expanded combinatorial libraries without any great loss. The one combinatorial library is packaged into phage particles and later used to infect the other combinatorial library (Fig. 2.8). Two plasmids now exist in the infected bacteria, which together code for the genetic information for the anchoring of a complete Fab molecule on the phage surface. Initially, only the genetic information for one of the two chains would be stored in the phage particle, because only one of the plasmids can be packaged into the phage particle. With the help of a recombinase (*cre* or *int*), this, too, can be achieved (Geoffroy et al., 1994; Griffiths et al., 1994). The recombination sequences that are recognized by cre, also serve in this instance as peptide linkers. As such, recombining the variable domains with each other into one scFV fragment is now possible (Tsurushita et al., 1996). This technique allows complexities to be achieved that exceed the phage number that can be used practically during screening. However, there is still room for improvement in this system. The recombination systems apparently impede bacterial growth, so that an increased number of mutations appear.

The *in vivo* new combination of both variable regions is a possibility offered by bacterial display vectors and has not yet been fully exploited (e.g., Fuchs et al., 1991; Francisco et al., 1993). As described above, at first, two combinatorial libraries can be constructed and enlarged millionfold. In this case, the genes of the antibody chains no longer need to be linked with a recombinase because the two plasmids are enriched together with the bacterium. The complexity of such a library is only experimentally limited by the number of bacteria that can be handled. Using the currently available techniques, complexities of 10^{16} independent clones can be achieved. It must be borne in mind that the efficiency of the selection systems is a further limitation factor. Until now, the screening

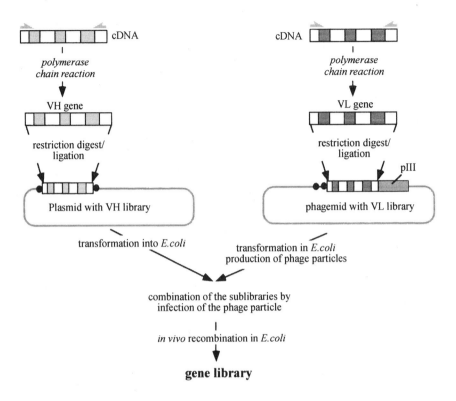

Fig. 2.8. The *in vivo* recombination of V region gene repertoires of the heavy and light chain in *E. coli*. For recombinant antibodies, the complexity of the antibody library is limited by the bottle neck of transformation. The complexity of recombinant antibody libraries can be multiplied by the combination of two combinatorial libraries. Thereby, the genetic information from two different plasmids is combined into a single phagemid by the activity of a recombinase. The resulting phagemids can then be packaged into phage particles, linking the (combined) antibody gene with Fab fragment presented on the surface of the phage. See Figure 2.7 for symbols; filled circles: recombination signals.

systems for bacterial display systems are not comparable to those for phage antibody systems. In the near future, however, the completion of very efficient selection instruments for these systems, which can manage a minimal complexity of 10^9 independent clones, is likely.

2.3 From Diversity to Specificity: The Selection of Recombinant Antibodies From Gene Libraries

The previous section discussed how the antibody diversity of the human body can be transferred into a bacterial system, and possibly even surpassed. The great diversity of antibody genes at first exists in the form of PCR bands or in the ligated plasmid vectors before they are transformed as efficiently as possible into bacteria. An antibody library is now the recognized term for this diversity. The selection systems used to isolate the desired antibody from this great diversity is the topic of the next section.

2.3.1 SELECTION OF RECOMBINANT ANTIBODIES WITH CLASSICAL EXPRESSION SYSTEMS

At the beginning, antibody libraries were screened using the classical techniques. As many *E. coli* colonies as possible (or plaques for a *lambda* phage cloning vector) are transferred to a filter and then screened for any antibody-binding activity (Huse et al., 1989). These techniques proved to be so successful that a human antitetanus antibody was discovered. The successors of this antibody may eventually be of use in the passive immunization against tetanus.

A similar detection system uses two nitrocellulose filters on top of one another. The bacterial colonies (the antibody library) are located on one filter and secrete an individual scFV fragment. All the scFv fragments that diffuse out from the bacterial colonies carry a small peptide at their C terminus (a *tag* or flag; see Section 4.4.4.2). This peptide anchors to the second filter that was previously incubated with an antibody against the peptide. An affinity purification of the scFv fragment is said to occur. In this way, the background of nonspecific signals is considerably reduced, and clones that produce the desired antibody can be identified by means of the antigen binding (Skerra et al., 1991).

All these detection systems are only suitable for small antibody libraries, in which only a few million clones can be analyzed by antibody binding. Larger numbers present the experimenter with insoluble technical problems, such that he or she literally drowns in a sea of filters and antigens that these types of selection systems require. This means that the great diversity of antibody genes, which can be obtained by the methods presented in Section 2.2, cannot be used to its full advantage by such selection systems.

2.3.2 GENES COUPLED TO THEIR GENE PRODUCTS

A very elegant solution for this selection problem is offered by the physical coupling of a gene and its gene product, a trick used by the B-lymphocytes of the immune system for millions of years (briefly described in Chapter 1, Figure 1.4). They present a membrane-bound antibody on their surface and the subsequent binding of an antigen (e.g., a virus) stimulates the B-lymphocyte to divide. The whole process is called *clonal selection*. The prerequisite for this clonal selection is the physical coupling of the antibody gene with its gene product, the antibody. Expressed differently, the antibody is said to carry its gene piggyback. For this type of selection, in principle, a single cell is sufficient to filter out the desired antibody producers from the myriad irrelevant B-lymphocytes.

If transferred to bacteria, this type of selection system would be vastly superior to those mentioned previously. This would mean that billions of different bacteria could be analyzed by antigen binding in a very small volume. The potentially very valuable antigen no longer needs to be applied in great quantities to nitrocellulose filters. In this case, the smallest amounts of antigen suffice to search for its specific binding partner. If the antigen is coupled to a solid phase, all the unbound cells can be washed away.

2.3.3 PEPTIDES CAN BE PRESENTED ON THE SURFACE OF BACTERIOPHAGES

In 1985, G. P. Smith succeeded in transferring this selection principle to filamentous bacteriophages. The life cycle of this group of phages (M13, fd, f1) is more precisely presented in Figure 2.9. They do not kill their host, *E. coli*, but instead slow growth by about half. Each bacterium releases 100–200 phage particles during one cell cycle. After infection via the F-Pili of the bacteria, the phage genome directs the replication of the phage DNA and the packaging of the single-stranded phage genome into long, filamentous particles. These very robust particles are exported into the culture medium from which they are easily purified.

Filamentous phage particles are very simply constructed. The genome of the phage comprises 6,500 bases of single-stranded, circular DNA surrounded by a tubulus of about 2,700 protein molecules of the gene product VIII (pVIII). The only additional components are five molecules each of pVII and pIX at one end and pIII and pVI at the other end of the filamentous phage particle (reviewed in Webster and Lopez, 1985; Rasched and Oberer, 1986).

Foreign peptide sequences can be integrated at different places in the pIII, without seriously impairing its function (Nelson et al., 1981; Smith, 1985; Parmley and Smith, 1988). In this way, the gene and its gene product are physically coupled. A direct consequence of this work enabled the production of peptide libraries, with which, for example, antibody-binding, peptide epitopes can be identified (Cwirla et al., 1990; Devlin et al., 1990; Scott and Smith, 1990). This surface expression or display vector is far superior to the membrane-bound selection systems. Up to 10^{14} phage particles can be concentrated into 1 ml and tested for binding. Simply all the unbound phage particles are washed away and those that bind are eluted. These are used to start a new infection cycle (screening round). In this way single phages can be found that lead to an antibiotic resistant bacterial colony, after a few hours of growth. It is this sensitivity that enables an enrichment of many orders of magnitude.

2.3.4 RECOMBINANT ANTIBODIES ANCHORED ON THE SURFACE OF FILAMENTOUS PHAGES

In 1990, an scFv fragment was first anchored on the surface of a filamentous phage, in the manner described above. This expression system, however, had

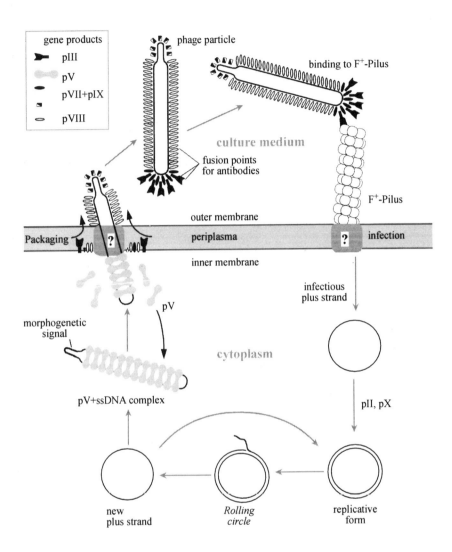

gene products
- pIII
- pV
- pVII+pIX
- pVIII

phage particle

binding to F$^+$-Pilus

culture medium

fusion points
for antibodies

F$^+$-Pilus

outer membrane

Packaging   ?   periplasma   ?   infection

inner membrane

morphogenetic
signal

pV

infectious
plus strand

cytoplasm

pV+ssDNA complex

pII, pX

new
plus strand

*Rolling
circle*

replicative
form

Fig. 2.9.   The life cycle of filamentous phages.

serious drawbacks for genes of size for antibody fragments (McCafferty et al.,1990). The bacteria were apparently poisoned by the corresponding phage particle, such that only a very poor production of these antibody phages was possible. The scFv fragment entailed a severe selection impediment for the corresponding phage particle. Figure 2.9 illustrates the possible reason for the poor production of these phage antibodies. The antibody pIII fusion protein must be expressed in each round of replication, because pIII is essential for phage infection. This causes a continual selection pressure against the fusion portions that impaired phage replication.

The use of phagemid vectors provided the breakthrough, because they mitigate the selection impediments (Barbas et al., 1991; Breitling et al., 1991; Hoogenboom et al., 1991). A phagemid (Fig. 2.10) is a completely normal plasmid that possesses an additional property. It includes a sequence of roughly

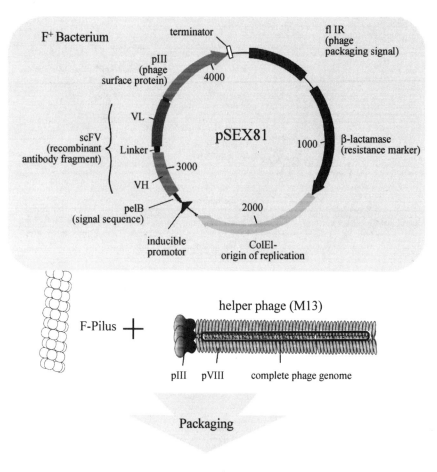

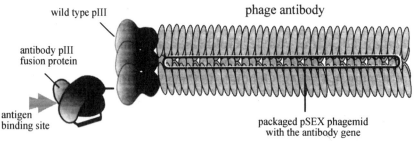

Fig. 2.10. Phagemids are plasmids that additionally possess a packaging signal a the filametous phages. (**Top**) In the presence of a helper phage, the phagemid DNA is packaged into a phage particle. (**Bottom**) Simultanous expression of the fusion protein scFv-pIII results in phage particles that display an antibody fragment on the surface.

500 bp of the phage genome that contains all the signals for the packaging of the phage particles. This phagemid DNA is assembled into normal phage particles by using a helper phage that directs all the other functions of the filamentous phage. Also in this case, the antibody fragment is anchored to the phage surface by fusion to the phage pIII coat-protein. This fusion protein is not constitutively expressed in the phagemid, as in the case above, but instead regulated externally under the control of an inducible promoter. Thus, the selection impediment described above is distinctly eased. The construction and amplification of the antibody library can take place without the expression of the antibody fragment, that is, without the concomitant selection impediment. The antibody–pIII fusion protein needs to be induced only for about two rounds of replication, while the helper phage is added simultaneously. Then, and only then, are phage particles formed that have an antibody fragment anchored to their surface, whose gene can now be selected because of the binding of this particle to the antigen. This is particularly advantageous when dealing with very large antibody libraries containing potential cloning artifacts. If the Fv–pIII fusion protein is constitutively expressed, the mutations that inevitably appear would dominate the library after a few rounds of replication.

2.3.5 BILLIONS OF DIFFERENT ANTIBODY CLONES CAN BE TESTED FOR BINDING WITH THE HELP OF DISPLAY VECTORS

Each phage particle described actually represents a very large molecular complex, and thereby fulfills the requirements of a physical particle that can be concentrated out from a suspension. A phage particle of this type can be bound to an immobilized antigen because of its surface-anchored scFv fragment, and can be enriched in a process that is analogous to affinity chromatography. First, the antibody library is packaged into phage particles by the addition of a helper phage. The expression of the recombinant antibody, fused to pIII, is induced only briefly, so that the selection pressure against successful recombination is reduced. The resulting phage particles, display their antibody fragments on the surface. Thus, by binding to antigen, they can be separated from unbound phages, which are washed away. In the next step, the phages are eluted with either acid or alkaline pH, or by trypsin. These enriched antibody phages can be used to infect new bacteria, which then produce the phage particle for the next round of selection. This enrichment is nothing other than the desired clonal selection.

Initially, chromatography material was still used for the enrichment (Breitling et al., 1991). Today, polystyrene plasticware (10-ml tubes or even ELISA plates) is used. The actual selection process is termed *panning*, borrowed from the gold-washing pans. The use of a biotinylated antigen is also possible, guaranteeing binding completely in solution. Bound phage particles are then separated and eluted from the remaining library with immobilized streptavidin (Schier et al., 1996).

This new method for expression screening has already proved its suitability for isolating new antibodies in numerous laboratories. Currently, the use of phagemid display vectors clearly dominates. References to individual examples are given in Section 2.2 on libraries. To date, the largest libraries described possess a complexity of ca. 10^{10} independent antibody genes (Nissim et al., 1994). Many antibodies have been selected from these libraries, even without prior immunization. A typical antibody selection is schematically presented in Figure 2.11. A comprehensive protocol for this type of selection can be found in Dörsam et al., (1997).

The biochemical conditions for the antigen incubation, washing and elution can be modified in several respects to influence the properties of the then selected antibodies, such as the *off-rate* or cross-reactivities. Differential screening is also possible, where first the unwanted specificities are removed and then desired antibody is sought in a subsequent round of screening (de Kruif et al., 1995a). This will be one of the most important applications of

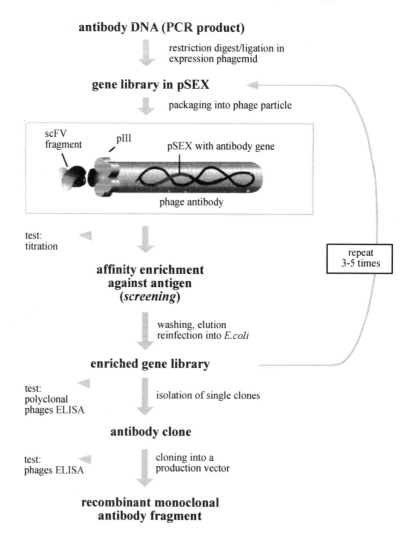

Fig. 2.11.   Selection of phage antibodies from an antibody library.

antibody libraries in the future, because the search then can be focused on the differences between two molecules or cells. An especially interesting question arises of whether new, tumor-specific antibodies can be successfully obtained in this way, which do not bind to the closely related precursor cells from which the tumor cells developed.

2.3.5.1 Affinity and Antigen Concentration are Important Parameters for Screening Highly Complex Antibody Libraries

The last few years have yielded a clear correlation between the success of the search for recombinant antibodies and the size of naive antibody libraries. The more complex the antibody library, the sooner recombinant antibodies of desired specificity could be isolated and the better these antibodies bound to their antigens. The most complex, naive, antibody libraries described to date comprise originally about 10^9 to 10^{11} independent transformants. All of these libraries are phagemid libraries. Here, the complexity lies close to the number of manageable phage particles.

Approximately 10^{13} phagemid particles per liter can be obtained from an overnight culture. A defined clone is then only represented roughly 1,000 times in a library with a complexity of 10^{10}. Moreover, a mixture of wild-type–pIII and antibody–pIII molecules are assembled on the surface as a result of using a wild-type helper phage for packaging. Therefore, at best some hundred functional antibody phages of a certain specificity can be obtained per liter of culture medium, from such a highly complex library.

This low number of specific antibody phages also means a lower probability that one of these particles actually exists bound to its antigen, which is made clear in the following numerical example. It is assumed that an antibody phage from the library binds its antigen with an affinity of 10^6 mol^{-1} l. The concentration of the antigen is taken as roughly 10^{-8} mol l^{-1} (e.g., 2 μg of a protein with a molecular mass of 200,000 Da in 1 ml). Put into the formula:

$$\frac{\text{concentration of the antibody phage bound to antigen (AB)}}{\text{concentration of unbound antibody phage (A)}} = \text{affinity constant} \times \text{antigen concentration (B)}$$

gives that $(AB) / (A) = (10^6 \text{ mol}^{-1} \text{ l}) (10^{-8} \text{ mol l}^{-1}) = 10^{-2}$. This means that in this numerical example, only *1 in 100* phages exists bound to its antigen. Thus, the probability is low that one of the few, originally utilized antibody phages survived the first round of selection. The screening of such a highly complex library is therefore very costly because, at least in the first selection round, either very large quantities of antibody phages or antigen must be utilized.

The quantity of antigen used in "panning" for selection can therefore determine the success of the screening or the properties of the selected antibody. In the simplest scenario, a large quantity of antigen (over 20 μg) is coupled to the plastic surface to tip the balance of the reaction in favor of the binding complex, despite the low number of potentially binding antibody phages. In other words, the use of low antigen concentrations runs the risk of losing existing antibody phages for kinetic reasons. This limitation also explains the initial lack of success in screening antibody libraries directly on cell surfaces, despite many attempts. The first successful isolation of recombinant antibody fragments occurred using phage display against cell surface antigens on red blood corpuscles, whose surfaces had a very high antigen density (Hughes-Jones et al., 1994).

These conditions can also be exploited. A reduction of the antigen concentration during screening, to a point where competition of the phage particles for the antigen can occur, those recombinant antibody fragments with the highest affinity can be preferentially selected (Schier et al., 1996).

2.3.5.2 Detection of Specifically Binding Antibody Phages

The first indication of whether an antibody fragment, isolated from a library, is really binding specifically is given by the number of phage particles that remain stuck to the immobilized antigen. This number can be determined by titration, and if it increases with each round of selection and only a few of the phage particles remain stuck to another antigen, these are good indications that the antibody phage is binding specifically to its antigen. A major advantage of this method is its extreme sensitivity. A phage particle, that is, a single molecule leads to a visible antibiotic resistant colony. A typical enrichment with antigen can be seen in Figure 2.12.

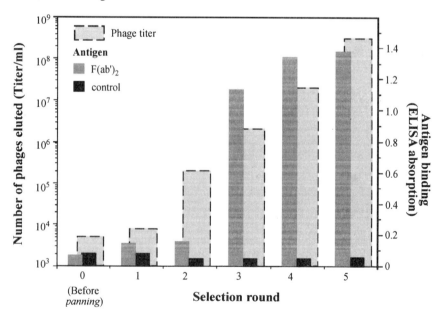

Fig. 2.12. The enrichment of phage antibodies using immobilized antigen. The increase in the number of phage particles bound to the antigen (titer) with each round of enrichment is shown. Simultanously, a comparative increase in antigen binding of the enriched phage particle fractions is demonstrated by phage ELISA. Antigen-specific antibody phages are detected with an antibody against the pVII phage coat protein that produces a color reaction. (Reproduced with the kind permission of M. Welschof and P. Terness.)

Phage-ELISA provides additional and more reliable evidence about the specificity of an enriched phage antibody. As with a normal ELISA, the antigen is immobilized on a plastic surface. After the saturation of nonspecific binding (blocking), phage antibodies derived from a single clone, or from a mixture, are applied and the nonbinding phages are washed away. The phage particles can be detected with a serum against the phage that, upon binding, leads to a colorimetric reaction. Usually more specific, is detection with a monoclonal antibody against the pVIII of the phage surface (Micheel et al., 1994), which is meanwhile commercially available. Due to the existence of pVIII in thousands of copies, the resulting signal is considerably amplified. The sensitivity of this phage ELISA yields a detection limit of $10^6 - 10^7$ phage particles and, therefore, is extraordinarily high. Apart from an ELISA, antibody phages can be used for a range of other immunological detection reactions such as immunoblotting and immunofluorescence.

To monitor the success of an enrichment, a "polyclonal" ELISA can be performed on aliquots of the total phage preparations, before and after each panning. This allows a determination, without the analysis of single clones, of whether a significant proportion of the specifically binding phage exists in the mixture (Fig. 2.12). If a clear signal is observed, 96 individual clones are cultivated in a deep-well plate (1 ml per well) and phage antibodies are produced with the addition of helper phage. The phage antibodies can be transferred into a second ELISA plate and tested for antigen binding. The selected clones are then subcloned into expression vectors to produce larger quantities of the recombinant antibody fragment. Detailed instructions for all these experiments are given in Dörsam et al., (1997).

2.3.6 DISPLAY VECTORS SIMPLIFY THE SELECTION OF HUMAN RECOMBINANT ANTIBODY FRAGMENTS

Selection systems such as display vectors simplify the development of human therapeutic agents because alternative methods, such as the established hybridoma technology, are only rarely available for the production of human antibodies. This is because human hybridoma cells are unstable compared to mouse lines, and keeping them in culture over extended periods is very difficult. As human antibodies are not recognized as foreign by the human immune system, they are of great interest especially for therapeutic applications. They can repeatedly be used as therapeutic agents, while the foreign mouse antibodies are quickly neutralized by the human immune system through the human-anti-mouse antibody (HAMA) response.

2.3.6.1 Recombinant Antibody Fragments Can Neutralize Viruses

For many viral illnesses there are still no antibiotics available comparable to penicillin, which today has reduced the dread of many bacterial infection diseases. A person must either be immunized in time, if the appropriate immunization exists, or he must trust in his immune system. The latter can very quickly become dangerous, especially in immunosupressed individuals (e.g., AIDS or kidney transplant patients) or in newborns. Patients who have just recovered from a viral infection are of great interest to the genetic engineers. Antibodies can be detected in the blood serum of these patients, which neutralize the viruses in cell culture systems. These antibodies are of great clinical interest because they could prove to be valuable therapeutic tools. They can be obtained as recombinant antibody fragments using the screening systems described in Section 2.3.4. The antibody genes of an individual who has successfully overcome a viral infection are subcloned by using a display vector. Those recombinant antibodies that bind to the virus particles can then be investigated for their neutralizing effects in a cell culture system. Sometimes the antibodies hinder the fusion of several infected cells; in other cases they hinder lysis. The proportion of neutralizing recombinant antibodies can sometimes be increased with a little trick. In the selection of the phage antibody just described, antibodies (monoclonal antibodies or another serum) that bind to the virus, but do not neutralize it, are added. In this way the epitopes that are not relevant in neutralizing the virus are obscured, and the search can be focused on those recombinant phage antibodies that bind the neutralizing epitope (Sanna et al., 1995). With this method, neutralizing recombinant antibodies against a multitude of viruses have since been discovered (Wiliamson et al., 1993), including RSV, HSV types 1 and 2, CMV, and HIV. Antibody fragments against HSV, RSV, and HIV have already proved their neutralizing effects in animal models (Crowe et al., 1994; Parren et al., 1995; Sanna et al., 1996). Recombinant antibodies against rubella, varicella zoster, and measles also exist. However, these either did not have a neutralizing effect in cell culture or, as for hepatitis B, still no cell culture model exists (Zebedee et al., 1992).

Recombinant antibodies do not have to be restricted to those against human pathogens. Of special interest is the fight against plant viruses. Transgenic commercial plants that express a neutralizing antibody fragment would confront the plant virus with a novel situation. For the first time the virus has to contend with a form of specific immune system. The first step in this direction can be viewed in terms of the self-production of recombinant antibodies directed against *cucumber mosaic cucumovirus* (Ziegler et al., 1995).

2.3.6.2 Recombinant Antibodies Against Autoantigens

Normally, only a few plasma cells that produce antibodies circulate in the blood. If autoreactive B-lymphocytes are activated, or high-affinity autoantibodies are formed, this can lead to autoimmune diseases. These are defined by the recognition and attack of the body's own structures by the immune system, for example type 1 (juvenile) diabetes or systemic lupus erythematosus, which are often fatal. In these patients, and also in those with HIV infections, a whole range of autoantibodies is usually detectable in the blood serum. For the first time, by using recombinant methods obtaining human monoclonal antibody fragments from the blood of these patients is possible (with certain exceptions). From the corresponding patient gene libraries, a host of autoantibodies has already been isolated. Examples include antithyroglobulin antibodies or anti-DNA antibodies (Hexham et al., 1994; Barbas et al., 1995), with whose help it may one day be possible to protect the body's own structures from attack by its own immune system.

A few publications have shown that looking to the antibody genes of autoimmune patients is not always necessary. Autoantibodies can be isolated also from normal, universal, antibody libraries, including recombinant antibodies against integrins with the astonishingly high affinity of 10^{-10} M (Barbas et al., 1993). Perhaps the reason for this success lies in the random new combination of the light and heavy chains during the construction of these antibody libraries. In contrast to the human immune system, which filters out, or at least suppresses the expression of these "self" antibodies during its development, the corresponding autoantibodies can be produced in bacteria.

Autoantibodies also exist that practice important regulatory functions in the immune system. An oligoclonal anti-Ig antibody, which each human possesses, serves as an example. This autoantibody probably participates in the regulation of the B-cell response (Süsal et al., 1992). An interesting finding was discovered in patients with autoimmune hemolytic anemia. Large quantities of the anti-Ig antibody in the blood serum correlate with low titers of the pathogenic antierythrocyte antibody and the other way round. This probably means that the autoreactive B-lymphocytes are suppressed by the anti-Ig antibody (Terness et al., 1995). Recently, an scFv fragment with these binding properties was cloned (Welschof et al., 1997a). The hope exists that one day a derivative of this recombinant antibody fragment will reduce the production of autoantibodies in autoimmune diseases, and that it can be used as a new type of immunosuppressive agent.

2.3.6.3 Antibodies of Therapeutic Interest

Particular interest is paid to tumor-associated antibodies for the treatment of cancer. A few such antibodies have already been isolated. They often recognize embryonic antigens, which, at least, are more often expressed on tumor cells than in normal tissues. One of these antibodies recognizes the carcinoembryonic antigen (CEA). The scFv fragment binds its antigen, CEA, with an especially high affinity (Chester et al., 1994). This scFv fragment will soon be tested for its suitability in the treatment of intestinal cancer. Antibodies against differentiation antigens like CD19 (on B-lymphomas) can also be used to fight tumors because the differentiated B-lymphocytes, for instance, can be replaced by stem cells from the bone marrow.

Another incentive to the search for tumor-associated antigens and the corresponding recombinant antibody fragments is based on the therapeutic success in intestinal cancer. This was made possible with an unconjugated monoclonal mouse antibody (Holz et al., 1996). A few recombinant, humanized antibodies are also already in clinical trials. An example is the humanized anti-TAC antibody (CAMPATH-1H) that is being used in the fight against T-cell leukemias (Hale et al., 1988). Other recombinant antibodies are being tested for their efficacy in animal models (Tsunenari et al., 1996); further examples are discussed in Chapter 3. Other therapeutically desired effects can also be communicated by recombinant antibodies, for example, they can be used as receptor antagonists where the control of activation is desired. An example is a scFv fragment that can suppress the cytotoxicity of tumor necrosis factor (TNF) (Moosmayer et al., 1995).

2.3.7 ANTIGEN-SPECIFIC INFECTION OF BACTERIA

An antigen-specific infection would mean a very elegant improvement of the selection system. In such a system, the survival of the phage would depend on its ability to infect bacteria, with the aid of its antibody portion. This can be achieved when the pIII molecule on the phage surface is divided into two parts. The portion that binds the F-Pili is produced in soluble form and coupled to the antigen. The portion anchored in the phage particle is fused to the recombinant antibody fragment. Reassembly of the complete pIII only occurs when the recombinant antibody fragment binds to the antigen (Fig. 2.13b). Only now can the phage particle infect its host bacterium. This has been accomplished (Duenas and Borrebaeck, 1994; Krebber et al., 1995), but with very low efficiency. This low efficiency is based on several factors. First, three different reaction partners must come together. For the molarities in complex libraries indicated above, this means that the binding partners only very rarely meet. Second, pIII possesses an extremely high affinity for the F-Pili. Therefore, the soluble pIII can only be used in very small quantities. Otherwise, it immediately saturates all the F-Pili. It seems that these are subsequently retracted into the bacteria — a very efficient form of competitive inhibition. Once more, this means that only very low concentrations of both binding partners can be used, that is, very few infection events take place. This method is thus not suitable for use in screening highly complex libraries. It could prove itself to be a good system for improving the affinity of recombinant antibody fragments, as the number of infection events is directly proportional to the affinity.

The above-mentioned limitations could be overcome by the direct fusion of the antigen with proteins of the F-Pilus (Rondot et al., 1998). In this case, only two binding partners are necessary and competition through soluble pIII does not occur because the system would not require it (Fig. 2.13c).

2.3.8 OTHER PROKARYOTIC DISPLAY VECTORS

Other expression vectors were also developed that guaranteed the desired linkage of a defined antibody specificity with its gene in a physical particle. For instance, an antibody fragment can be anchored to the cell wall of *E. coli* (Fuchs et al., 1991). Analogous to the B-lymphocyte, the antibody is situated on the surface of the bacterium, inside which the gene for this antibody is carried. An antibody-displaying bacterium can be colored with a fluorescently labeled antibody and later separated from nonfluorescent bacteria with the aid of a *fluorescence-activated cell sorter* (FACS) (Francisco et al., 1993; Fuchs et al., 1996).

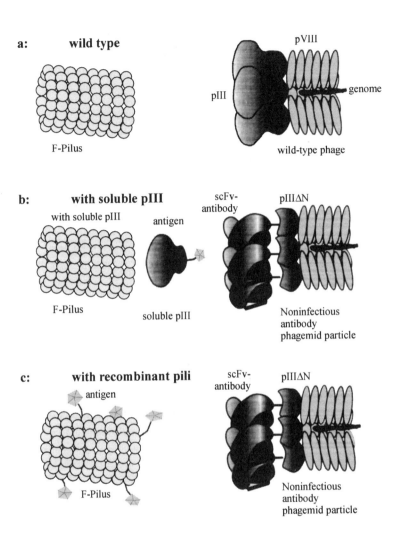

a: wild type

F-Pilus

pVIII

pIII

genome

wild-type phage

b: with soluble pIII

with soluble pIII

antigen

F-Pilus

soluble pIII

scFv-antibody

pIIIΔN

Noninfectious
antibody
phagemid particle

c: with recombinant pili

antigen

F-Pilus

scFv-antibody

pIIIΔN

Noninfectious
antibody
phagemid particle

Fig. 2.13. Antigen-dependent infection (*in vitro* evolution) (**a**) The wild-type phage binds with the complete pIII to the F-Pilus. This leads to infection. (**b**) The N-terminal moiety of the phage surface protein pIII (ΔCpIII), is produced in a soluble form by the replacement of the carboxyterminus with antigen. Thus, it mediates the binding between pilus and phage antibody. Only antibody phages that specifically bind to the antigen can infect bacteria. (**c**) When the antigen is directly incorporated into the pili, the ΔCpIII can be omitted. The production of phagemid particles that no longer possess wild type infection ability is a prerequisite for panels b and c. This is ensured by the use of pIII without an amino terminus (antibody-ΔNpIII fusions).

Apart from the bacterial display vectors, there are also a few, further phage coat proteins that serve as anchors for recombinant proteins. For the filamentous phages, apart from the pIII described above, the coat proteins pVI and pVIII have been used as fusion anchors for foreign peptides. The pVIII molecule occurs as a few thousand copies on the phage surface, while only five representatives each of pIII and pVI are to be found on the phage surface. pVIII, however, is unsuitable for the anchoring of antibody fragments. Despite the intensively practiced phage genetics, no mutations of pVIII exist that result in viable phage particles. This means that pVIII fusions can only be used in a mixture with wildtype pVIII. Therefore, it is not possible to control if, and in what quantities, the pVIII-antibody fusion protein is assembled in the phage particle (Kang et al., 1991). Until now, only peptides have been fused to the pVI coat protein of filamentous phages (Jespers et al., 1995). The potential of this system in screening antibody libraries must still be investigated. Recently, a display vector based on T7 phages has been described (Rosenberg et al., 1996). This system is probably not suitable for antibody fragments because the T7 phages are assembled in the cytoplasm. This is the wrong compartment for the construction of antibody fragments because the reducing conditions here do not allow the formation of the disulfide bridges, which normally are essential for antibody folding.

2.3.9 ANTIBODIES CAN ALSO BE ANCHORED ON THE SURFACE OF EUKARYOTIC VIRUSES

Antibodies can also be displayed on the surface of recombinant eukaryotic viruses. Often, this occurs with the goal of constructing a specific vehicle for somatic gene therapy. The antibody is supposed to provide the specificity that allows it to transform only certain cells (Russell et al., 1993). Eukaryotic viruses have also been used for screening an antibody library. A library from the spleen of immunized mice was inserted into baculoviruses. Antitetanus toxoid antibody fragments were isolated successfully from this library (Ward et al., 1996). The advantage of the eukaryotic systems lies especially in the existence of a folding apparatus, which is much more suitable for the functional expression of antibody fragments than that of *E. coli*. Obtaining antibodies from such systems that can only be produced in insoluble forms in bacteria should be possible. At present, a methodological drawback of eukaryotic systems however, is the limited number of transformants that can be attained. Therefore, the use of highly complex antibody gene libraries is ruled out. The above-mentioned library contained only 2×10^4 independent clones. Additionally, the costs and the experimental sterility requirements are higher than those for bacterial systems. Therefore, the use of these systems should remain limited to very specific queries, where the use of bacteria is not possible.

2.4 Antibody Engineering

2.4.1 WHY ANTIBODY ENGINEERING?

The first two sections dealt with the construction of antibody libraries and the appropriate screening systems. This section is about improving antibodies, in the widest sense. Improvement can concern specificity, affinity and the produceability in heterologous organisms like *E. coli*. It can also mean that the specificity of an antibody is widened to include several antigen variants. The reverse can be helpful when, for example, the specificity of a tumor specific antibody is narrowed and thus less healthy tissue is destroyed as a result. For many applications, it is not sufficient only to improve the affinity of an antibody. In a few applications, particularly small antibody fragments are necessary, mouse antibodies must be changed into human ones, or the folding or protease stability of an antibody must be increased.

An example should make this clear. The starting point may be a monoclonal mouse antibody that binds specifically to a solid tumor. This would be an ideal candidate for a highly specific tumor therapy, when the antibody is used as a toxin transporter (immunotoxin), for example. The complete antibody often does not fulfil its expectations because it is too large to diffuse far enough into the tumor. Thus, it must be made smaller. The best candidate would be the smallest antibody fragment that could still bind the antigen, the Fv fragment of this antibody. The Fv fragment, however, is not stable enough. The antibody transporter and its toxin cargo would break apart before it can unload its fatal cargo in the tumor. Therefore, it must be stabilized first. Additionally, the affinity of the antibody should be as high as possible because the better the antibody binds to its antigen, the tumor, the less dangerous cargo is mistakenly transported through the body, and the more likely the antibody will reach its goal. But this is of no help, if the immune system of the patient decides to recognize this mouse antibody as foreign because, after a few days, the human anti-mouse antibodies bar the way to the target, the tumor. To solve this problem, genetic engineering accomplished the technical requirements to make it possible to alter antibody genes and to select them based on their desired properties. Today, a variety of plasmid vectors allow the expression of antibody genes in the most diverse cell lines. Thus, a great breakthrough was certainly the first production of larger quantities of functionally competent antibody fragments in *E. coli*. This is because refined techniques for this organism are meanwhile available with which antibody fragments with completely new properties can be sought (Better et al., 1988; Skerra and Plückthun, 1998).

2.4.2 MOUSE–HUMAN CHIMERAS

A plethora of mouse hybridoma antibodies of potential therapeutic interest is already available. A problem for their therapeutic use is their mouse origin because proteins from a foreign species are recognized as foreign by the human immune system (Courtenay Luck et al., 1986; Lamers et al., 1995). This results in the formation of the HAMA immune response. These antibodies are formed within a few days by the human immune system, and, normally, they neutralize the therapeutically administered mouse antibodies and render them inactive (Fig. 2.14). The possibility of repeat therapy is therefore very limited.

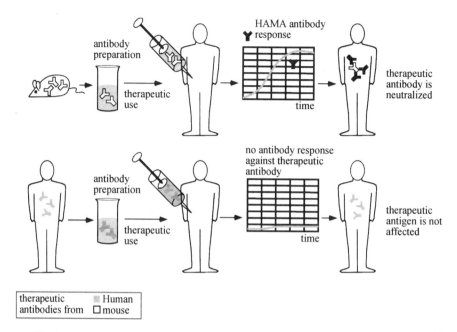

Fig. 2.14. HAMA (*human anti-mouse antibodies*) are formed by the human immune system as a response against therapeutic or diagnostic mouse antibodies. Therefore, the mouse antibodies are neutralized after a few days and rendered ineffective. The use of humanized antibodies for therapeutic or diagnostic purposes drastically reduces this immune response.

Most of the HAMA antibodies are directed against the constant portion of the mouse antibodies. This provided the incentive for the production of *antibody chimeras*. A term borrowed from Greek mythology, these are the antibody genes mixed together from two, different life forms. A variable, mouse antibody domain is followed by the constant antibody domain from humans (reviewed in Wright et al., 1992). First, a human antibody gene is placed into a cloning vector. The individual antibody domains form compact, folded units which are connected to each other with a peptide strand. The exchange of whole antibody domains keeps the chance of a disruption in antibody function to a minimum. Today, with the invention of the polymerase chain reaction, it is no problem to produce chimeric cDNAs, because precise cloning has been distinctly simplified with this technique. The resultant chimeric antibodies (Fig. 2.15) still bind specifically to the antigen, however the HAMA response is clearly reduced. The constant domains now stem from man, and thus, these chimeric antibodies activate some helper functions of the human immune system distinctly better, such as the antibody-dependent cellular cytotoxicity (ADCC). This is a further reason why a few such humanized antibodies are already found in clinical trials (reviewed in Winter and Harris, 1993).

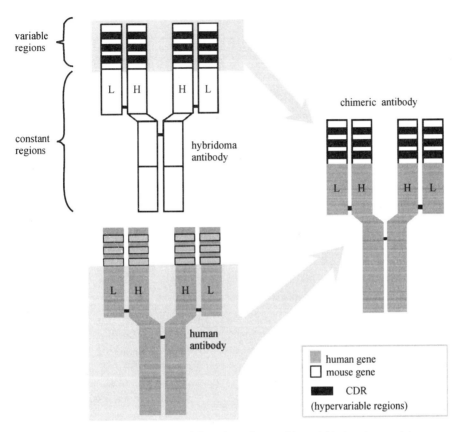

variable regions

constant regions

L H H L

hybridoma antibody

human antibody

chimeric antibody

L H H L

L H H L

human gene
mouse gene
CDR
(hypervariable regions)

Fig. 2.15. Chimeric antibody genes result from the exchange of the variable domains - a mixture of genes from two different species. Thus, the constant (larger) portion of existing, clinically interesting, mouse antibodies can be humanized and thereby made invisible to the human immune system. In this way, a large portion of the HAMA antibodies (see Fig. 2.14) can be avoided.

2.4.3 FRAMEWORK REGIONS OF THE VARIABLE DOMAIN FROM MOUSE ANTIBODIES CAN BE HUMANIZED

The *humanization* of antibodies, described in the previous paragraph, strongly reduces the HAMA response but a few HAMA antibodies are also formed against the remaining mouse portion, the variable domains. These domains can be categorized into the hypervariable domains (*complementarity determining regions* [CDRs]) and the framework regions that are less variable (see Section 1.1.2). Compared to the hypervariable areas, these framework portions are conserved. There are a limited number of framework areas coded for by a family of closely related genes. This led to the notion of transferring the hypervariable regions of a mouse antibody into a related human framework area, to bring about CDR *grafting* (Fig. 2.16). The first attempts of this type led to antibodies whose affinity for the antigen was distinctly lower than that of their predecessor, the mouse antibody. Along with the rapidly expanding knowledge of the three-dimensional structure of many different antibodies, the

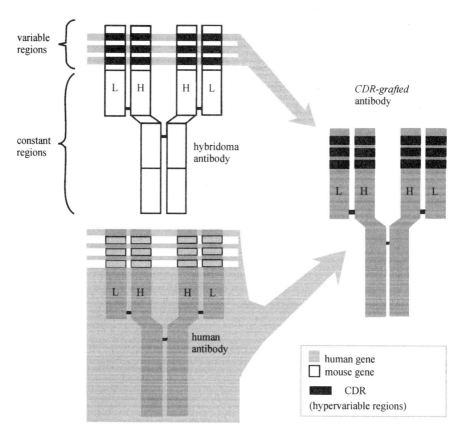

Fig. 2.16. A fully humanized antibody results from the grafting of the hypervariable areas of a mouse antibody. Apart from these hypervariable domains, nothing else could be recognized as "foreign" by the human immune system.

results of the CDR exchange also improved. Nowadays, the affinity of several fully humanized antibodies can hardly be distinguished from the parental mouse antibody (Riechmann et al., 1988; Foote and Winter, 1992; Studnicka et al., 1994). With these antibodies the HAMA should no longer play a role in the therapeutic usage in humans.

These studies also provided some fundamental discoveries about the importance of certain amino acids in the variable domains of the antibody. It is known today that some amino acid pairs are irreplaceable for the stability and correct folding of the variable domains. The heavy, variable domains of subgroup III require, for example, a phenylalanine partner at position 67 for the glycine at position 9. In the other subgroups, the amino acids proline, alanine or serine at position 9 correlate with a nonaromatic amino acid at position 67 (Saul et al., 1993). The size of the amino acid at position 71 determines which from five various conformations the CDR II of the VH domains will take (Tramontano et al., 1990). Some other amino acids anchor the hypervariable areas into the framework regions. These amino acids cannot be altered in the humanization of the antibody.

2.4.4 THREE-DIMENSIONAL STRUCTURE OF ANTIBODIES CAN BE MODELED ON A COMPUTER

The humanization of antibodies could not have been accomplished without the availability of X-ray crystallography data, which permitted precise statements about the three-dimensional structure. To date, many different antibodies have been crystallized (Braden et al., 1995). Investigation of the alpha C atom, that is, the backbone of the antibody structure, showed that the framework regions fold themselves into a few forms that are very similar to each other. Surprisingly, this was also true for most of the CDRs that can be similarly organized into corresponding *canonical structures* (Chothia et al., 1992). Until now, a consensus structure cannot be defined for only the amino acid loop, coded for by the third hypervariable area of the VH domain. The loop coded for by the first hypervariable area of the VH domain, folds itself into one of three possible consensus structures, while the second hypervariable area codes for one of five different consensus structures. The combination of these consensus structures would yield 15 different spatial structures for the arrangement of the two first hypervariable loops of the VH domain alone. Until now, only seven of these combinations have actually been found. Maybe the other combinations are sterically hindered. Perhaps, it is also not at all necessary to proffer all the possibilities. The structures used might have been sufficient for evolution to construct the antibody diversity. A recent study also included the known spatial consensus structures of the three CDRs of the light variable domain. The basis was 381 known antibody sequences. From the 300 possible consensus structures, only 29 were discovered. The majority (87%) of examined antibodies were related to 1 of only 10 of these 29 structures (Vargas-Madrazo et al., 1995).

This makes the antibodies ideal candidates for understanding the principles of protein folding because a limited number of consensus structures simplify the structure prediction. It has always been a dream of many molecular biologists to be able to predict the three-dimensional structure (and function) of a protein from the protein sequence. The hypervariable regions offer a model system that allows the structural prediction to be experimentally checked relatively easily. Currently, there are computer programs that have proved their accuracy in predicting the folding of the various hypervariable areas (Roberts et al., 1994; accessible on the WWW site, http://www.biochem.ucl.ac.uk/~martin/antibodies.html). The first published structural prediction, for example, correctly predicted the structure of the framework area from four of the six hypervariable areas (Chothia et al., 1986).

Many successful experiments meanwhile are based on antibody models from a computer. For example, with their help, Fv fragments were stabilized through additional disulfide bridges (Brinkmann et al., 1993) (see Section 3.2). The computer models show their worth often in conjunction with experimental data about the three-dimensional structure. NMR can help in the identification of the amino acids of the Fv fragments that participate in antigen binding, because binding to antigen specifically reduces the degrees of freedom of the amino acids involved. With this knowledge, a computer model was compiled of a scFv fragment bound to its antigen, phenyloxazolone. From this structural prediction, a single amino acid was changed, causing the affinity of the scFV fragment to be increased threefold (Riechmann et al., 1992). This rational design could prove to be very useful in the future, where improving the specificity or the affinity of a Fv fragment is concerned.

The most comprehensive attempt in this direction, is the *de novo* modeling of a complete antigen binding site on a computer. Schiweck and Skerra (1997) constructed an antibody against cystatine purely based on crystal structure data. This endeavor required several steps in the approach to the desired structure, each of which were checked by the crystallization of the antibody–antigen complex. In the future, it may be possible to use the knowledge thus obtained to design antibodies against antigens that cannot be achieved the natural way, for example, when the antigen is highly toxic. Therefore, computer modeling will possibly be available in the future as an alternative to screening of display libraries. The prediction of the binding affinity of an antibody to its antigen however, is still a long way off, because the smallest deviation in the structural prediction can cause large differences in the binding to antigen. Moreover, problems with the expression in *E. coli* may seriously retard such a design plan.

2.4.5 EFFICIENT SCREENING SYSTEMS HELP IN THE HUMANIZATION OF ANTIBODIES THROUGH *CHAIN SHUFFLING*

The approach described in the previous section, assumes a good knowledge about the three-dimensional structure of the antibody. It is not so apparent that a good knowledge about the dynamics of the protein folding is also necessary. The rational design too often fails and although the antibody is humanized, it is no longer correctly folded or does not bind to its antigen any more. An alternative humanizing strategy is offered by the efficient screening systems introduced in Section 2.3. They allow an evolutionary approach, in which a functional antibody is chosen from many different possibilities. First, the mouse antibody is expressed as the Fv or Fab fragment in phage selection vectors. In the next step, the gene for the light chain (and in a parallel experiment, the gene of the heavy chain) is exchanged for a library of human antibody genes. Phage antibodies, which still bind the antigen, are then pursued (Fig. 2.17). This method is called *chain shuffling*. If the light and heavy chains found in this way are put together, or if this process is carried out for both V regions in turn, a humanized antibody is obtained that should bind the same epitope as the mouse antibody from which it descends (Jespers et al., 1994).

2.4.5.1 Mouse Antibodies Focus the Search for Humanized Antibodies on the Original Epitope in *Chain Shuffling*

An interesting variation of this humanizing strategy is *chain shuffling* on a protein level. The starting points are human phage–antibody libraries that,

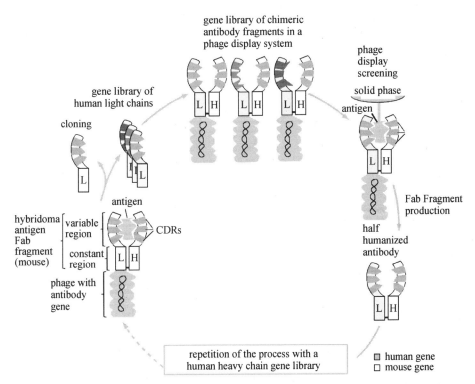

Fig. 2.17. Humanization of antibodies by chain shuffling. Using a display system, millions of phage antibodies can be simultaneously screened for antigen binding. When one of the V regions of the original antibody is held constant, the search for humanized antibodies is focused upon the original epitope. The figure illustrates humanization of the light chain of a Fab fragment as an example. The heavy chain can be humanized in the same way as the light chain. The combination of both chains then leads to a complete human Fab fragment.

this time, do not carry any complete Fab fragments on their surfaces but only the part of the Fab fragment coded for by the heavy chain. In this approach, the *protein* of the mouse hybridomal antibody is used instead of the gene, to find out its human equivalent. First, the hybridomal antibody is reduced. This dissolves the disulfide bridges that stabilize the connection between the light and heavy chain (Fig. 2.18). The light chain is later mixed with the phages of the human combinatorial library. Under oxidizing conditions, a large number of newly combined Fab molecules are formed that are all displayed on a phage surface. From these combinations, the phages are sought that bind to the same antigen as the mouse antibody. In this way, the human gene for a heavy chain is at hand. In the next step, this heavy chain is joined with a combinatorial library from human light chains and so, a complete humanized Fab fragment is obtained (Figini et al., 1994). This strategy obliviates the construction of a recombinant mouse antibody and its expression in bacteria. Instead of the arduous reconstruction of the hybridomal antibody into a recombinant mouse antibody, here falling back on existing availabilities is possible: the antibody protein and two human antibody combinatorial libraries.

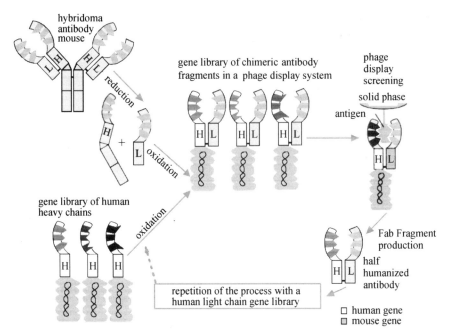

Fig. 2.18. Humanization by chain shuffling on a protein level. Instead of the arduous construction of a new recombinant mouse phage antibody from the genes of the hybridomal antibody, the hybridoma protein is used here to find the humanized antibody. Once again, one antibody chain is held constant so that the search for humanized antibodies is focussed on the original epitope. The humanization of an Fab fragment heavy chain is shown as an example in this figure. The light chain can also be humanized with an Fv fragment paralleling the humanization of the heavy chain. The combination of both chains then leads to a complete human Fab fragment.

2.4.6 AFFINITY OF RECOMBINANT ANTIBODIES CAN BE INCREASED BY REPEATED MUTATION AND SELECTION

The techniques just described not only allow the antibody to be humanized but also can be used to increase its affinity for the antigen (Figini et al., 1994). Again, the example set by nature can be followed. In our immune system, the variants that bind the best dominate over the assortment of randomly generated variants. The deciding factor is that many antibodies must compete for little antigen. This is usually easy to manage experimentally. A large number of phage antibodies must simply compete for little antigen. In this way, it can even be decided whether the affinity, or only the dissociation constant, of the phage antibody should be improved. In the first case, the phage antibodies are allowed to compete for a low amount of biotinylated antigen. The number of antigen molecules should exceed the number of phage antibodies, but the concentration of the antigen should be somewhat below the dissociation constant. Thus, predominantly mutated phage antibodies with increased affinity bind to the biotinylated antigen, while the larger part of the weaker affinity phage antibodies remains unbound.

Streptavidin then can assist in the enrichment of the higher affinity, mutated phage antibodies from the mixture (Schier et al., 1996). For some therapeutic applications, slowing the dissociation from the antigen in particular is desirable. For example, this applies to an antibody that should concentrate in tumor tissues over many days. To achieve this, the phage antibodies are first bound to biotinylated antigen and then an excess of unbiotinylated antigen is added. After sometime, predominantly the phage antibodies with the lower dissociation constant can be harvested with streptavidin (Hawkins et al., 1992).

The prerequisite for this is the largest possible number of antibody variants from which a selection can then be made. The immune system guarantees this through somatic hypermutation (see Section 1.1.7). Genetic engineers have developed many techniques to bring about the corresponding mutations in the test tube. First, the *chain shuffling* described above can be conducted. Here, a library from different light or heavy chains can be used that can lead to the variants that bind with higher affinity. The affinities of various antibodies were increased up to 20-fold using this method (Marks et al., 1992).

Even closer to the example set by nature is the use of a mutator strain, that is, an *E. coli* cell line with a strongly elevated mutation rate. A mutant with a hundredfold increased affinity for the antigen was isolated from phagemid antibodies passaged through this strain (Low et al., 1996). It remains to be seen if this can succeed as a routine method because the increased mutation rate can lead to technical problems.

2.4.7 ANTIBODY GENES CAN BE MUTATED WITH GENE SYNTHESIS OR WITH THE HELP OF THE POLYMERASE CHAIN REACTION

Mutations can also be selectively inserted into the antibody gene, for example, with the help of the PCR. Experimental conditions are chosen in which the error rate of the polymerase is artificially increased in the assembly of nucleotides, for example, with suboptimal salt concentrations (Fig. 2.19). The mixture of the mutated antibody genes is then again put into a display vector and screened for phage antibodies that bind better, as described above. This protocol is actually very close to nature's example in that it starts with an already binding antibody, whose affinity is improved merely through small changes (Hawkins et al., 1992).

Alternatively, the antibody can be mutated only in its CDR regions (Barbas et al., 1994; Deng et al., 1995). The methodology for this has already been introduced in Sections 2.2.8 and 2.2.9. The CDR regions are replaced with random sequences from synthetic oligonucleotides. An especially impressive improvement in the affinity was achieved in this way in an HIV-1 neutralizing antibody. First, only the CDR I area of the VH domain was exchanged for random nucleotides. Then, the mutated antibody genes were screened for better binding variants with the help of a display vector. In the next step, the CDR III area of the VH domain was exchanged for random nucleotides. Again, screening for the variants that bound the best was performed and this process

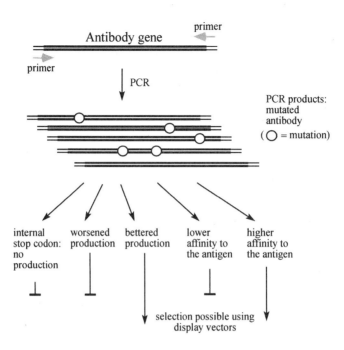

Fig. 2.19. Random mutations can be introduced into antibody genes with the help of the polymerase chain reaction. The resultant mutants with the desired properties can be selected from a large number of mutated antibody genes using surface expression. This selection yields antibodies that are better produced by the bacterium or have a higher antigen affinity.

was repeated with three further CDRs. This yielded several different recombinant antibodies that bound the antigen up to ninety-six times better than the starting antibody. The next question was then, if the combination of some of these mutations could improve the affinity of the antibody for its antigen still further. This was generally not so, but for one of the combinations of several mutations, an improved affinity of 420 times that of the starting antibody was determined. The antibody affinity, achieved in this way, of 15pM for its antigen gp120, is remarkable. This type of high affinity antibody is found extremely seldom in nature (Yang et al., 1995). Such a combination of various mutations is, however, a very arduous undertaking. The workload to produce all the possible combinations of only twenty different mutations is already very large. Therefore it is better to limit the somatic hypermutation to a few prudent amino acids in the (already functional) antibody gene. In this way, the chance exists, right from the start, to isolate high affinity antibody fragments from the antibody library. The reason for this is that probably many combinations of prudent (i.e., affinity-increasing) mutations already exist in this library, while otherwise the chance that two random mutations inside the antibody gene contribute to an increase in affinity is extremely low.

Which amino acid residues should be mutated to increase the affinity of this antibody for its antigen? Naturally the first candidates are the amino acid residues that participate in antigen binding. First, the amino acid residues that participate in antigen binding must be identified, for example, with the help of NMR (see Section 4.1.1). The codons for these can be exchanged with random sequences using oligonucleotides. Then, a phage antibody library can be screened for the antibodies that bind the best. Using this technique, the affinity of a scFv fragment for its antigen phenyloxazolone could be increased 11- to 15-fold (Riechmann and Weill, 1993). This so-called semirational design combined structure prediction, three-dimensional information from NMR and surface expression to improve the affinity of a Fv fragment.

2.4.8 "SEXUAL" PCR COMBINES SEVERAL MUTATIONS

With the methods described in the previous chapter, a diversity of antibody variants can be obtained that then must be arduously combined with each other. The combination of two variants, that each may have a higher affinity, in no way necessarily leads to a still further improved Fv fragment. On the contrary, that is only rarely the case. There is, however, one possibility to combine many mutations in one simple experiment. It has already been discussed above that random mutations can be inserted into the antibody genes by the polymerase chain reaction. If, for example, the mutation A now exists in a DNA molecule after the fifth cycle, this mutation is passed down to its descendants formed in the following cycles. Normally, this mutation would not be combined with another mutation B, which, exists in another DNA molecule after the seventh cycle. This mutation is also passed down to the next generations, so that after 20 cycles, many molecules with mutation A exist and concurrently, many molecules with mutation B. It is however, very improbable that one of the antibody genes carries both mutations because until now, all the mutations were separately passed down to the next generations. Evolution has found a very successful solution for this repeatedly occurring problem: sexual recombination. A prerequisite for the imitation of a corresponding new combination of mutations, *in vitro*, is first a fragmentation of the DNA molecules. A few cuts per DNA molecule are made by DNase I that is, each DNA strand is fragmented. The fragments with the different mutations are not yet intermixed, but after heating and then cooling, the different fragments are randomly hybridized to each other, that is, a recombination occurs. Then the PCR, which was interrupted by the DNase I digestion, is continued for a few cycles (Fig. 2.20). Therefore, this method is also called "sexual" PCR or "molecular breeding" (Stemmer, 1994). The mutated and intermixed antibody genes can thereby form complete antibody genes, in which now all the mutations were randomly mixed together. After cloning into a display vector, the so-produced gene library can be screened, as described above, for higher affinity or better produced antibodies.

Combining already existing antibody variants with each other would be easier still, of course. The sexual PCR just described, is then simply conducted with a mixture of DNA from the previously selected antibody variants (see previous section). This protocol has a very big advantage because it builds upon already improved antibody fragments. In this way, the number of purposeful combinations is largely increased in comparison to the combinations from

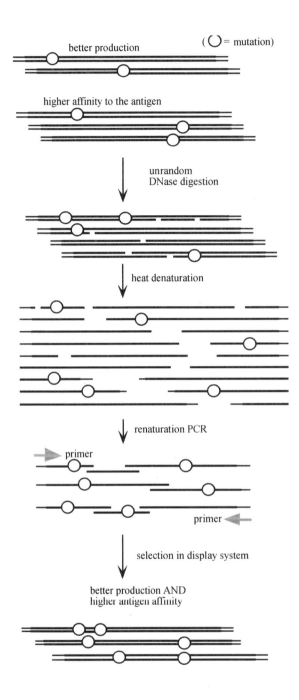

Fig. 2.20. Several mutations within a gene can be randomly combined using "sexual" PCR or "molecular breeding". The gene is fragmented by the action of the enzyme DNaseI. Heat denaturation followed by hybridization yields a novel combination of different fragments. These are repaired and amplified by the continuation of the PCR. The desired, altered properties of the gene can be then sought with an efficient screening system.

random mutations. A higher affinity antibody is more likely to be discovered from a library such as this, than from a library made up from combinations of random mutations that were not preselected.

2.4.9 Fv FRAGMENTS ARE STABILIZED THROUGH A PEPTIDE BOND LINKING THE VARIABLE DOMAINS

Fv fragments are only half as large as the corresponding Fab fragment and many times smaller than an IgG (see Figs. 1.1 and 1.2). This size difference is the deciding advantage of the Fv fragment in many applications. Smaller molecules, for example, can enter deeper into a solid tumor because the entry depth is usually limited, in this case, by diffusion. Conversely, the Fv antibodies are so small that they are filtered out by the kidneys. The two facts together are desirable for tumor detection by immunoscintigraphy (detailed in Section 3.3.3). Many Fv fragments are not very stable, their two component units, the VH and the VL domain, dissociate easily. The published affinity of the two variable domains for one another is scattered over a wide range between 10^{-5} mol/l to 10^{-8} mol/l (Glockshuber et al., 1990). The reason for this is probably that natural immunoglobulins do not require any additional stabilization by the variable domains. They are sufficiently stabilized through the binding of the constant domains to each other and through an $S = S -$ bridge between the light and heavy chain. Therefore, the artificial Fv fragments must be additionally stabilized. A possibility for this exists, because the variable domains of the heavy and light chain can be connected with each other with the help of a short peptide. In this way, a *single chain* antibody, scFv, is formed. A pleasant side effect of this is that one gene results from the two genes of the light and heavy chains. This eases the transfection of a functional antibody fragment into eukaryotic cells. The danger no longer exists that the light and heavy chains integrate at different places in the genome or that later, different amounts of the corresponding proteins are formed. The expression of similar quantities of both regions in *E. coli*, is also guaranteed.

Existing data on the three-dimensional structure of many antibody fragments show that the peptide linkers, in a scFv fragment, must span a distance of 35–40 Å. Thus, the distance from the C terminus of the VH domain to the N terminus of the VL domain is somewhat shorter than the reverse, the C terminus of the VL domain bound to the N terminus of the VH domain. Based upon this structural data, very different peptide linkages have been published meanwhile, usually with a length of 15–20 amino acids (Bird et al., 1988; Huston et al., 1988). Longer linkers are also possible. A natural linker peptide of 28 amino acid residues that flexibly binds the two domains of the *Trichoderma reesei* cellobiohydrolase I, has been successfully used to connect VH and VL regions (Takkinen et al., 1991). In other studies, a minimum length of only 12 amino acids was determined (Pantoliano et al., 1991; Alfthan et al., 1995), or a *tag* (see Section 4.4.4.2) was inserted into the linker (Breitling et al., 1991). All these peptide linkages yield functionally competent scFv antibody fragments, actually an astounding result, considering the relatively large distance between the N and C termini. The NMR data, and the successful structural determination of a scFv fragment, show that the amino acids in the peptide links between the variable domains are very flexible. They could not be fitted to any clear, fixed, three-dimensional structure (Raag and Whitlow, 1995). In one case, however, the insertion of a linker into an Fv fragment reduced its affinity for antigen two-threefold (Mallender et al., 1996).

The search for higher affinity scFv fragments, using phage display yielded a surprising result. After the selection, it was observed that, of the phage antibodies that bound better, several had a very short peptide bond between the variable domains. These Fv antibodies could no longer fold as a monomer due to the now, too short peptide link. Instead each two of them formed a dimer. The reason for the selection of these so-called "diabodies" was the doubling of the binding sites, and the resultant increased apparent affinity for the antigen, arising from avidity effects (see Section 4.1.2.7) (Schier et al., 1996). This is discussed further in Section 3.2.2.1.

The diabodies lead to a great problem in the production of scFv fragments. Many laboratories have since reported that scFv fragments aggregate at high concentrations (1–5 mg/ml). The reason for this aggregation is obviously the usually low affinity of the VH and the VL domains for each other. As such, the majority of the scFv fragments possess reaction-competent variable domains, that is, the VH domain of one scFv fragment can lie with the VL domain of another scFv fragment, resulting in the formation of dimers, oligomers and finally, insoluble aggregates.

This aggregate formation can sometimes be reduced by the addition of antigen, L-arginine, low pH values or low temperature. This still remains a serious problem however. scFv fragments cannot be highly concentrated. Their production is arduous and the specificity of antigen recognition is reduced by the unspecific deposition of aggregates. A comparison of peptide links of different lengths (15 aa, 20 aa, 25 aa, 30 aa) showed that the longer peptide links formed significantly fewer dimers than the 15 aa linkers (Raag and Whitlow, 1995).

Another way to reduce this problem is the use of the phage display systems described above. Beyond being able to find higher affinity antibody fragments with this system, improved production and solubility in *E. coli* are also being selected simultaneously. When a mutation improves the production and solubility of the scFv fragment in *E. coli*, this mutated scFv fragment has a higher probability of being displayed on the surface of a phage. Under suitable selection conditions, these antibody phages dominate over their forerunners. In one example, the effects of mutating Ile77 in the VH domain to a threonine caused the production of the scFv fragments in *E. coli* to increase by a factor of 10, and at the same time, the solubility increased by fourfold. In contrast, the affinity of the mutated scFv fragment remained unchanged (Deng et al., 1994). More suitable linker sequences can be discovered using such a screening system. Instead of a defined DNA sequence, random oligonucleotides are built in between both of the variable domains of a known Fv fragment. Finally, the scFv antibody phages with the best solubility, the lowest tendency to aggregate and also, of course, the best affinity can be selected with the help of antigen (Stemmer et al., 1993). Apparently, there are many equally good options for the choice of linkers in *E. coli*, however. Hardly any limitations in the possible sequences were found in possibly the most comprehensive study, apart from a conserved proline at the second position from the end of heavy chain (Tang et al., 1996).

2.4.10 Fv FRAGMENTS CAN BE STABILIZED THROUGH INTERNAL DISULFIDE BRIDGES

Although the scFv fragments are more stable than Fv fragments without stabilizing linkers, they are still vastly inferior to a Fab or even IgG in this respect. Their half-life in blood is about 2 hours at 37°C, compared with more than 14 hours for the corresponding Fab fragment or several days for the IgG antibody. This is much improved when the Fv fragment is stabilized with an internal disulfide bridge instead of a peptide linker. This disulfide bridge is inserted into the interphase between VH and VL, by the exchange of other amino acids for cysteine at this position (Fig. 2.21). The thus formed, dsFv fragments (ds for disulfide-stabilized) usually differ little from a Fab fragment in terms of half-life (reviewed in Brinkmann, 1996).

The dsFv fragments are, in other respects, astoundingly stable molecules. They require 7 mol/l urea to be irreversibly denatured, compared to less than 0.5 mol/l for the corresponding scFv fragment. The improved stability of the dsFv fragments has a range of less obvious consequences. They do not aggregate as readily as the scFv fragments, and as such, the yield of these fragments is usually increased in *E. coli* (Reiter et al., 1994). This property is

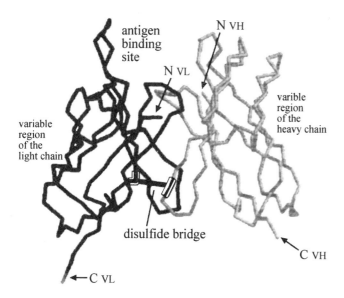

Fig. 2.21.   dsFv antibody fragments. A disulfide bridge can be used to stabilize the Fv fragments instead of a peptide link between the two chains of the variable domains. dsFv fragments in the bloodstream, stabilized in such a way, are similarly stable to the corresponding Fab fragments. This property is of great use for therapeutic applications.

still more important in the therapeutic or diagnostic application of these dsFv fragments. Here, aggregated antibodies would be usually very disruptive, because as a rule, the specificity of the antibody fragment is reduced. In tumor therapy, this means that a fatal cargo could be unloaded at the wrong place.

Knowledge about the three-dimensional structure of antibodies also helped in the construction of dsFv fragments. The distances between the individual amino acids, inside the fully folded antibody, can be measured exactly for some antibodies that have resolved crystal structures. With this information, some amino acids could be identified that, when changed into cysteines, have exactly the right distance from each other to form $S = S$ – bridges (Glockshuber et al., 1990). Using structure predictions, even conserved amino acid positions inside the framework regions have been discovered. When exchanged for cysteines, they have stabilized each antibody tested through an internal disulfide bridge (Jung et al., 1994; Reiter et al., 1994). Eight different dsFv fragments are compared with the corresponding scFv fragments in Table 2.2. In two cases, the affinities of the dsFv fragments were clearly lower and in another two cases they were about the same. Surprisingly, however, the affinity for antigen was increased in four of the tested scFV fragments by the inclusion of a disulfide

Table 2.2   Comparison of the Affinities of Eight different dsFv fragments with the corresponding scFv fragments, Fab fragments and IgGs

Antibody	Specificity	Construct	Affinity (nM)
B3	Lewis$^{\gamma}$	IgG	200
		Fab	1,400
		scFv-PE38	1,300
		d sFv-PE38	24,000
B1	Lewis$^{\gamma}$	IgG	100–200
		scFv-PE38	1,000
		dsFv-PE38	4,000
Anti-Tac	IL2R	IgG	1,2
		scFv-PE38K	1,4
		dsF v-PE38K	1,1
e23	erbB2	IgG	3
		Fab	8
		scFv-PE38K	40
		dsFv-PE38K	10
55.1	Mucine carbohydrate	IgG	3
		scFv-PE38	120
		dsFv-PE38	80
HB21	Transferrin receptor	IgG	20–25
		scFv-PE38KDEL	20–25
		dsFv-PE38KDEL	20–35
Y10	Mutated EGFR	IgG	10
		scFv-PE38K	450
		dsF v-PE38K	150
RFB4	CD22	IgG	10
		scFv-PE38	90
		dsFv-PE38	10

Reiter et al. (1996).
The scFv and dsFv fragments used were, in this case, fused to various versions of the *Pseudomonas* exotoxin.

bridge. This shows that the smallest shifts in the protein framework can lead to large changes in the affinity of the antibody.

2.4.11 CAMEL ANTIBODIES CONTAIN ONLY ONE VARIABLE DOMAIN

Over several decades, there have been repeated reports that the VH domain alone is sufficient for antigen binding (Utsumi and Karush 1964; Ward et al., 1989). This is more rarely described for the VL domain alone. In principle, shortening the Fv fragment even more should thus be possible. Some research groups were, indeed, successful in this effort, but usually the shortened antibody fragments were relatively insoluble. This led to aggregation and thus, nonspecific binding. In the most radical attempt to date, a VH domain was shortened to 61 amino acids, that is, in comparison to the Fv antibody, not only the VL domain was missing, but also the CDR3 and the framework 4 of the VH domain. These "minibodies" were mutated and their solubility improved by using the previously described phage display particles. Then, the CDR1 and the CDR2 regions were exchanged for random stretches and an interleukin-6 antagonist was isolated from the resulting phagemid library (Pessi et al., 1993; Martin et al., 1994).

Again, nature had already performed a similar experiment long ago. Most of the antibodies from camels and their relatives possess only one variable domain. The variable domain of the light chain is totally absent. The CH1 domain of the heavy chain is also deleted (Hamers-Casterman et al., 1993; Desmyter et al., 1996). Despite this, the camel obviously possesses functional antibodies of sufficient diversity. Producing universal binding molecules that are only half the size of the already small Fv fragments must therefore be actually possible. This binding fragment also should not be recognized by the human immune system as foreign, that is, it should be as similar to human antibody sequences as possible. These considerations were the starting points for the construction of a VH phagemid display library. Here, only the human VH domains are displayed on the surface of the phage particles. The VL domain is totally absent. Specifically binding antibody fragments, against a range of antigens such as lysozyme or the hapten phenyloxazolone, were indeed discovered from such a library, using the screening procedures described in Section 2.3.5. Apart from their specific binding, all these VH fragments also bound nonspecifically, especially to hydrophobic substances. The region that normally serves to bind the VL domain was responsible for this nonspecific binding activity of the VH fragment (Davies and Riechmann, 1995).

A comparison with the camel antibodies, in which the VL domain is naturally absent, was of help. Some amino acids, which in human VH domains establish contact with the VL domain, were mutated in the VH domain of the camel. Usually, a hydrophobic amino acid was changed into a hydrophilic amino acid. Yet more differences exist. In the CDR3 of the camel VH domain, the salt bridge between Arg 94 and Asp101 is missing. It is particularly striking that the CDR3 region of the camel is considerable more heterogeneous in comparison to human sequences. The length of the region varies to a much greater extent and moreover, a cysteine is often found in the CDR1 as well as in the CDR3. These two cysteines can form a supplementary disulfide bridge, which additionally stabilizes the expanded antigen-binding site of the camel VH domain (Muyldermans et al., 1994; Desmyter et al., 1996; Spinelli et al., 1996).

All these differences were taken into consideration in the construction of a camellike, human VH domain library. Several antigen specific VH fragments were isolated from some 2×10^6 different VH fragments displayed on the surface of filamentous phages. These fragments showed hardly any nonspecific binding. Moreover, they were astoundingly stable, losing their binding activity only at temperatures around 72°C (Davies and Riechmann, 1996). Next to the above mentioned "minibodies," these fragments currently represent the smallest, known, universal, human binding molecules. Due to their small size, they could gain great importance one day, especially in the treatment of solid tumors.

2.4.12 ANTIBODIES CAN TAKE OVER THE FUNCTION OF ENZYMES

Many years ago, Linus Pauling had already postulated that antibodies, in principle, should be able to take over the function of enzymes, namely, in a reaction from state A to state B, they could stabilize the transition state of a molecule by binding to it (Fig. 2.22). Of course, an enzyme or a catalytic antibody can only accelerate reactions that liberate energy. They reduce the activation energy required by the reaction (Schultz and Lerner, 1995).

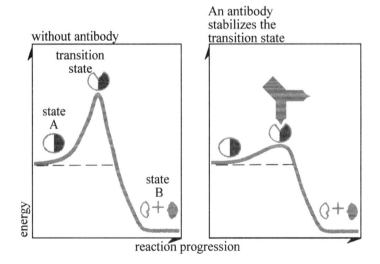

Fig. 2.22.   Antibodies can take over the function of enzymes. They stabilize the transition state of a reaction and thus lower the required activation energy to achieve this transition state. In this way, they accelerate the course of the reaction.

Enzymes (and catalytic antibodies) can reduce the activation energy in different ways, for example, they can aid the molecule in deciding which of many possible reaction routes it should follow. What does this decision-making aid look like on a molecular level? An organic molecule usually has many possibilities for how to order its atoms in three-dimensional space. Additionally, this ordering continually changes due to brownian motion and molecular oscillations. Only a few of these conformations will enable the reaction of a molecule to proceed in a certain direction, that is, at a given time point, only a few molecules are able to follow this reaction route. Binding to a partner strongly limits the number of possible conformations, because in many of the possible conformations, the binding partner is in the way and energy must be spent to dissolve this bond. Enzymes or catalytic antibodies as binding partners, preferentially impair the conformations that prevent the reaction of the molecule from proceeding to state B. By contrast, as few conformations as possible, that allow a reaction, are obstructed. In this way alone, they increase the rate of the reaction, often considerably.

A second possibility is to clear the way for the reaction. A catalytic antibody (or enzyme) offers the molecule an alternative route, for example, in which the molecule (and the antibody itself) is slightly altered. It then uses the free energy, which is liberated in the reaction, to resume its former conformation.

Once the desired reaction has occurred, the catalytic antibody should be able to leave the end product as quickly as possible, so that the reaction cycle can start again with a new molecule right away. This step determines the turnover-rate of the reaction.

How can those antibodies with catalytic activity be found from the many billions of different antibodies that exist? The working principles, already stated by L. Pauling, pointed out the way. He postulated that antibodies with catalytic activity stabilized the transition state of a reaction (Fig. 2.22). If a likeness of the transition state is successfully synthesized, as exact and stable as possible, a mouse can probably be immunized with it. The immune system of the mouse then forms antibodies against this transition state. The desired catalytic antibodies should be found among these (Lerner et al., 1991). A prerequisite for this, naturally, is that the transition state is known and that an analogue can be synthesized.

Often, nature provides the clue, for today it is known that many enzyme inhibitors mimic the transition state of the catalyzed reaction. The enzyme binds with high affinity to the inhibitor that, in contrast to the substrate, is not released and thereby blocks the enzyme activity. After a mouse was immunized with the inhibitor of the enzyme ferrochelatase, it actually formed catalytic antibodies with ferrochelatase activity (Cochran and Schultz, 1990). One of the obtained, monoclonal antibodies had a catalytic activity that is quite comparable with the corresponding enzyme.

The technology of recombinant antibodies has also made an advance into catalytic antibodies (Gibbs et al., 1991), which could accelerate the arduous search for catalytic antibodies in the future. In the mean time, enzymes were displayed on the surface of phages and enriched with the aid of a suicide inhibitor, by virtue of their catalytic activity (Soumillion et al., 1994). In another attempt, phagemid antibodies were sought that were bound with the substrate via a disulfide bridge. The phagemid antibodies were then eluted with the reducing agent DTT. The feat here, was that actually no free SH- groups were available at all in the substrate, and thus, the existing disulfide bridges in the substrate must have been broken first, a catalysis must have occurred (Janda et al., 1994). Perhaps in the future, there will be catalytic antibodies that, following a similar principle, will react with very reactive substrates and thereby "refuel" energy. They could then use this energy to catalyze reactions that, without them, would not continue voluntarily. This is very similar to many reactions that take place in cells, which only proceed with the concomitant hydrolysis of ATP (Wirsching et al., 1995).

Considerably more elegant, is the combination of the recombinant antibodies through positive selection, where the catalytic antibody helps the bacteria or yeast to survive. To date, two functional model systems have been described for this. A catalytic antibody was expressed in the cytoplasm of yeast that split the precursor chorismate into prephenate, which is necessary for the biosynthesis of the aromatic amino acids phenylalanine and tyrosine. The catalytic antibody takes over the job of the enzyme chorismatmutase (EC 5.4.99.5), which is defective in this yeast strain. In this way it helps the yeast strain, which is auxotrophic for the synthesis of these amino acids, to grow on a medium that is deficient in these amino acids (Tang et al., 1991).

A catalytic scFv antibody, expressed in *E. coli*, functions according to the same principle. It replaces the enzyme orotidine-5'-monophosphate decarboxylase (OMP, EC 4.1.1.23). This enzyme is essential for pyrimidine synthesis. The specific activity of the catalytic scFv antibody was about ten millionfold worse than the activity of the OMP-decarboxylase, but it was still about a hundred millionfold above background. This catalytic activity was sufficient to allow the bacterium to survive on a pyrimidine-deficient medium (Smiley et al., 1994).

Currently, already more than 60 different reaction paths can be accelerated by catalytic antibodies, including exotic catalyses such as cocaine hydrolysis (Landry et al., 1993). In the future, a humanized form of this catalytic antibody could treat acute cocaine poisoning. Catalytic antibodies can also be used in tumor therapy, in that they convert a relatively nontoxic precursor into a toxic molecule at the site of the tumor. This principle is described more precisely in Section 3.3.2.5. Two model systems currently exist: First, mustard gas is split out from a precursor by a catalytic antibody (Wentworth et al., 1996) and second, the antibiotic chloramphenicol is formed (Miyashita et al., 1993). The great advantage of a catalytic antibody, at least potentially, is its human origin, which differentiates it from the bacterial enzymes otherwise used.

Why is there, additionally, such a great interest in catalytic antibodies? To date, they can achieve catalytic rates that are, at best, comparable to the corresponding enzyme, but the surpassing of enzymes, which have been optimized over billions of years of evolution, will probably not be successful. The answer lies in the fact that evolution had only to find a limited number of catalysts. Therefore, there are no catalysts for many interesting reaction pathways. Antibodies, however, should also be able to catalyze new and "unnatural" reaction pathways. Thus, there is hope for new types of catalytic activities. They could, e.g., specifically inactivate viruses or disintegrate the

Alzheimer peptide. They could enable new types of syntheses in organic chemistry, which could lead to microprocessors a thousandfold smaller, or that neutralizes toxic substances in the blood.

A few small steps into this future have already been taken. There are, indeed, catalytic antibodies that enable new types of catalysis. A specific peptide synthesis serves as an example (Hirshmann et al., 1994; Jacobsen and Schultz, 1994). Perhaps one day, there will also be a specific peptide hydrolysis through catalytic antibodies, which could simplify biochemical analyses. Antibodies with serine protease activity have already been described (Zhou et al., 1994).

The work of Hollfelder and coworkers (1996) should serve as a sobering experience. They report that simple bovine serum albumin catalyzed a reaction as equally well (or better: equally badly) as a previously published catalytic antibody. Additionally, a further limitation exists in the synthesis of the transition state. Not all reactions are well enough understood that the transition state can be defined. Often, this is also impossible from a purely technical stand point — the transition state is known but there is no way to synthesize a stable molecule that resembles it.

Surprisingly, it was recently made known that naturally occurring antibodies could also have catalytic activity. It has long been known that the autoimmune disease systemic lupus erythematosus (SLE) correlates with the appearance of DNA-binding antibodies. These anti-DNA antibodies often not only bind DNA but also hydrolyze it with a turnover rate that is comparable to restriction endonucleases like EcoRI (Shuster et al., 1992). Other naturally occurring catalytic antibodies hydrolyze naturally occurring peptides (Paul et al., 1989; Li et al., 1995). Still, the question remains what physiological relevance these catalytic antibodies possess.

2.5 Summary

The immune system of higher vertebrates has been performing antibody engineering for millions of years. Suitable antibodies are chosen from a huge number of antibodies formed randomly by the combination of building blocks. This process is called *clonal selection*. These antibodies are improved through subsequent rounds of selection. Mutations, which are randomly inserted into the antibody genes, lead to a few antibody variants that have improved binding. Memory cells that code for these improved binding antibodies, survive in the competition against cells that present variants on their surfaces that do not bind so well. This process is called *somatic hypermutation*.

Molecular biology has made use of these principles in antibody engineering. A large number of antibodies, formed according to the random principle, are anchored to the surface of bacteria or bacteriophages. A selection of the desired antibodies then takes place by their binding to the antigen. This process can be repeated. An intercalated mutation in the antibody genes, analogous to somatic hypermutation, leads to the selection of better-binding antibodies. With the help of this method, libraries that contain billions of different antibodies can be screened for the antibodies of choice.

Already existing mouse monoclonal antibodies of potential clinical interest, can be humanized in the same way for use in patients. Alternatively, this can be performed using *rational design*. This makes use of the wealth of knowledge about the crystal structure of many different antibodies. In this way, the framework of a mouse antibody can be exchanged for a similar human framework. This process is called *CDR grafting*. A great advantage of recombinant antibodies is the ability to manipulate them. They can be made smaller, the affinity can be increased, they can be stabilized through S = S bridges in the base framework of the variable domains and they can obtain new properties through fusion with other proteins. These altered antibody fragments have a great future in the diagnosis and therapy of diseases. They can neutralize viruses and toxic substances and detect tumors. Catalytic antibodies can practice the functions of enzymes. Most catalytic antibodies function by stabilizing the transition state.

References

Akamatsu Y, Cole MS, Tso JY, Tsurushita N (1993) Construction of a human Ig combinatorial library from genomic V segments and synthetic CDR3 fragments. *J. Immunol* **151**:4651–4659.

Alfthan K, Takkinen K, Sizmann D, Soderlund H, Teeri TT (1995) Properties of a single chain antibody containing different linker peptides. *Protein Eng* **8**:725–731.

Ames RS, Tornetta MA, McMillan LJ, Kaiser KF, Holmes SD, Appelbaum E, Cusimano DM, Theisen TW, Gross MS, Jones CS (1995) Neutralizing murine monoclonal antibodies to human IL 5 isolated from hybridomas and a filamentous phage Fab display library. *J Immunol* **154**:6355–6364.

Anderson PS, Stryhn A, Hansen BE, Fugger L, Engberg J, Buus S (1996) A recombinant antibody with the antigen-specific, major histocompatibility complex-restricted specificity of T cells. *Proc Natl Acad Sci USA* **93**:1820–1824.

Arkin AP, Youvan DC (1992) Optimizing nucleotide mixtures to encode specific subsets of amino acids for semi random mutagenesis. *Biotechnology* **10**:297–300.

Barbas CF III, Kang AS, Lerner RA, Benkovic SJ (1991) Assembly of combinatorial antibody libraries on phage surfaces: the gene III site. *Proc Natl Acad Sci USA* **88**:7978–7982.

Barbas CF III, Bain JD, Hoekstra DM, Lerner RA (1992) Semisynthetic combinatorial antibody libraries: a chemical solution to the diversity problem. *Proc Natl Acad Sci USA* **89**:4457–4461.

Barbas CF III, Languino LR, Smith JW (1993) High affinity self reactive human antibodies by design and selection: targeting the integrin ligand binding site. *Proc Natl Acad Sci USA* **90**:10003–10007.

Barbas CF III, Hu D, Dunlop N, Sawyer L, Cababa D, Hendry RM, Nara PL, Burton DR (1994) *In vitro* evolution of a neutralizing human antibody to human immunodeficiency virus type 1 to enhance affinity and broaden strain cross reactivity. *Proc Natl Acad Sci USA* **91**:3809–3813.

Barbas SM, Ditzel HJ, Salonen EM, Yang WP, Silverman GJ, Burton DR (1995) Human autoantibody recognition of DNA. *Proc Natl Acad Sci USA* **92**:2529–2533.

Better M, Chen CP, Robinson RR, Horowitz AH (1998) *Escherichia coli* secretion of an active chimeric antibody fragment. *Science* **240**:1041–1043.

Bird RE, Hardman KD, Jacobson JW, Johnson S, Kaufman BM, Lee SM, Lee T, Pope SH, Riordan GS, Whitlow M (1998) Single chain antigen binding protein. *Science* **242**:423–426.

Bornemann KD, Brewer JW, Beck Engeser GB, Corley RB, Hass IG, Jack HM (1995) Roles of heavy and light chains in IgM polymerization. *Proc Natl Acad Sci USA* **92**:4912–4916.

Braden BC, Poljak RJ (1995) Structural features of the reactions between antibodies and protein antigens. *FASEB J* **9**:9–16.

Braunagel M (1995) Konstrucktion und Screening einer synthetischen Antikörperbibliothek. Dissertation, Universität Heidelberg.

Breitling F, Dübel S (1997) Cloning and expression of single chain fragments (scFv) from mouse and rat hybridomas. Methods Mol Med.

Breitling F, Dübel S, Seehaus T, Klewinghaus I, Little M (1991) A surface expression vector for antibody screening. *Gene* **104**:147–153.

Brinkmann U (1996) Recombinant immunotoxins: protein engineering for cancer therapy. *Mol Med Today* **2**:439–446.

Brinkmann U, Reiter Y, Jung SH, Lee B, Pastan I (1993) A recombinant immunotoxin containing a disulfide stabilized Fv fragment. *Proc Natl Acad Sci USA* **90**:7538–7542.

Campbell MJ, Zelenetz AD, Levy S, Levy R (1992) Use of family specific region primers for PCR amplification of the human heavy chain variable region gene repertoire. *Mol Immunol* **29**:193–203.

Chester KA, Begent RH, Robson L, Keep P, Pedley RB, Boden JA, Boxer G, Green A, Winter G, Cochet O (1994) Phage libraries for generation of clinically useful antibodies. *Lancet* **343**:455–456.

Chothia C, Lesk AM, Levitt M, Amit AG, Mariuzza RA, Phillips SE, Poljak RJ (1986) The predicted structure of immunoglobulin D1.3 and its comparison with the crystal structure. *Science* **233**:755–758.

Chothia C, Lesk AM, Gherardi E, Tomlinson IM, Walter G, Marks JD, Llewelyn MB, Winter G (1992) Structural repertoire of the human VH segments. *J Mol Biol* **227**:799–817.

Cochran AG, Schultz PG (1990) Antibody catalyzed porphyrin metallation. *Science* **249**:781–783.

Cook GP, Tomlinson IM (1995) The human immunoglobulin VH repertoire. *Immunol Today* **16**:237–242.

Courtenay Luck NS, Epenetos AA, Moore R, Larche M, Pectasides D, Dhokia B, Ritter M (1986) Development of primary and secondary immune responses to mouse monoclonal antibodies used in the diagnosis and therapy of malignant neoplasms. *Cancer Res* **46**:6489–6493.

Crowe JE Jr, Murphy BR, Chanock RM, Williamson RA, Barbas CF III, Burton DR (1994) Recombinant human respiratory syncytial virus (RSV) monoclonal antibody Fab is effective therapeutically when introduced directly into the lungs of RSV infected mice. *Proc Natl Acad Sci USA* **91**:1386–1390.

Cwirla SE, Peters EA, Barrett RW, Dower WJ (1990) Peptides on phage: a vast library of peptides for identifying ligands. *Proc Natl Acad Sci USA* **87**:6378–6382.

Davies EL, Smith JS, Birkett CR, Manser JM, Anderson Dear DV, Young JR (1995) Selection of specific phage display antibodies using libraries derived from chicken immunoglobulin genes. *J Immunol Methods* **186**:125–135.

Davies J, Riechmann L (1995) Antibody VH domains as small recognition units. *Biotechnology* **13**:475–479.

Davies J, Riechmann L (1996) Single antibody domains as small recognition units: design and *in vitro* antigen selection of camelized, human VH domains with improved protein stability. *Protein Eng* **9**:531–537.

de Kruif J, Boel E, Logtenberg T (1995a) Selection and application of human single chain Fv antibody fragments from a semi synthetic phage antibody display library with designed CDR3 regions. *J Mol Biol* **248**:97–105.

de Kruif J, Terstappen L, Boel E, Logtenberg T (1995b) Rapid selection of cell subpopulation specific human monoclonal antibodies from a synthetic phage antibody library. *Proc Natl Acad Sci USA* **92**:3938–3942.

de Kruif J, van der Vuurst de Vrias AR, Cilenti L, Boel E, van Ewijk W, Logtenberg T (1996) New perspectives on recombinant human antibodies. *Immunol Today* **17**:453–455.

de Wildt RM, Finnern R, Ouwehand WH, Griffiths AD, van Venrooij WJ, Hoet RM (1996) Characterization of human variable domain antibody fragments against the U1 RNA associated A protein, selected from a synthetic and patient derived combinatorial V gene library. *Eur J Immunol* **26**:629–639.

Deng SJ, MacKenzie CR, Sadowska J, Michniewicz J, Young NM, Bundle DR, Narang SA (1994) Selection of antibody single chain variable fragments with improved carbohydrate binding by phage display. *J Biol Chem* **269**:9533–9538.

Deng SJ, MacKenzie CR, Hirama T, Brousseau R, Lowary TL, Young NM, Bundle DR, Narang SA (1995) Basis for selection of improved carbohydrate binding single chain antibodies from synthetic gene libraries. *Proc Natl Acad Sci USA* **92**:4992–4996.

Desmyter A, Transue TR, Ghahroudi MA, Thi MHD, Poortmans F, Hamers R, Muyldermans S, Wyns L (1996) Crystal structure of a camel single domain VH antibody fragment in complex with lysozyme. *Nature Struct Biol* **3**:803–811.

Devlin JJ, Panganiban LC, Devlin PE (1990) Random peptide libraries: a source of specific protein binding molecules. *Science* **249**:404–406.

Dinh O, Weng NP; Kiso M, Ishida H, Hasegawa A, Marcus DM (1996) High affinity antibodies against Lex and sialyl Lex from a phage display library. *J Immunol* **157**:732–738.

Dörsam H, Braunagels M, Kleist C, Moynet D, Welschof M (1997) Screening of phage displayed antibody libraries. Methods Mol Med.

Dübel S, Breitling F, Fuchs P, Zewe M, Gotter S, Moldenhauer G, Little M (1994) Isolation of IgG antibody Fv DNA from various mouse and rat hybridoma cell lines using the polymerase chain reaction with a simple set of primers. *J Immunol Methods* **175**:89–95.

Dübel S, Breitling F, Kontermann R, Schmidt T, Skerra A, Little M (1995) Bifunctional and multimeric complexes of streptavidin fused to single chain antibodies (scFv). *J Immunol Methods* **178**:201–209.

Duchosal MA, Eming SA, Fischer P, Leturcq D, Barbas CF III, McConahey PJ, Caothien RH, Thornton GB, Dixon FJ, Burton DR (1992) Immunization of hu PBL SCID mice and the rescue of human monoclonal Fab fragments through combinatorial libraries. *Nature* **355**:258–262.

Duenas M, Borrebaeck C (1994) Clonal selection and amplification of phage displayed antibodies by linking antigen recognition and phage replication. *Bio/Technology* **12**:999–1002.

Dziegiel M, Nielsen LK, Andersen PS, Blancher A, Dickmeiss E, Engberg J (1995) Phage display used for gene cloning of human recombinant antibody against the erythrocyte surface antigen rhesus D. *J Immunol Methods* **182**:7–19.

Embleton MJ, Gorochov G, Jones PT, Winter G (1992) In cell PCR from RNA: amplifying and linking the rearranged immunoglobulin heavy and light chain V genes within single cells. *Nucleic Acids Res* **20**:3831–3837.

Figini M, Marks JD, Winter G, Griffiths AD (1994) *In vitro* assembly of repertoires of antibody chains on the surface of phage by renaturation. *J Mol Biol* **239**:68–78.

Foote J, Winter G (1992) Antibody framework residues affecting the conformation of the hypervariable loops. *J Mol Biol* **224**:487–499.

Francisco JA, Campbell R, Iverson BL, Georgiou G (1993) Production and fluorescence activated cell sorting of *Escherichia coli* expressing a functional antibody fragment on the external surface. *Proc Natl Acad Sci USA* **90**:10444–10448.

Frippiat JP, Williams SC, Tomlinson JM, Cook GP, Cherif D, Le Paslier D, Collins JE, Dunham I, Winter G, Lefranc MP (1995) Organization of the human immunoglobulin lambda light chain locus on chromosome 22q11.2. *Hum Mol Genet* **4**:983–991.

Fuchs P, Breitling F, Dübel S, Seehaus T, Little M (1991) Targeting recombinant antibodies to the surface of *E. coli*. Fusion to a peptidoglycan associated lipoprotein. *Bio/Technology* **9**:1369–1372.

Fuchs P, Dübel S, Breitling F, Braunagel M, Klewinghaus I, Little M (1992) Recombinant human monoclonal antibodies: Basic principles of the immune system transferred to *E. coli*. *Cell Biophys* **21**:81–92.

Fuchs P, Weichel W, Dübel S, Breitling F, Little M (1996) Specific selection of *E. coli* expressing functional cell wall bound antibody fragments by FACS. *Immunotechnology* **2**:97–102.

Fuchs P, Breitling F, Little M, Dübel S (1997) Primary structure and functional scFv antibody expression of an antibody against the human protooncogene c myc. *Hybridoma* **16**:227–233.

Geoffroy F, Sodoyer R, Aujame LA (1994) New phage display system to construct multicombinatorial libraries of very large antibody repertoires. *Gene* **151**:109–113.

Gibbs RA, Posner BA, Filpula DR, Dodd SW, Finkelman MA, Lee TK, Wroble M, Whitlow M, Benkovic SJ (1991) Construction and characterization of a single chain catalytic antibody. *Proc Natl Acad Sci USA* **88**:4001–4004.

Glockshuber R, Malia M, Pfitzinger I, Plückthun A (1990) A comparison of strategies to stabilize immunoglobulin Fv fragment. *Biochemistry* **29**:1362–1367.

Gram H, Marconi LA, Barbas CF III, Collet TA, Lerner RA, Kang AS (1992) *In vitro* selection and affinity maturation of antibodies from a naive combinatorial immunoglobulin library. *Proc Natl Acad Sci USA* **89**:3576–3580.

Griffin HM, Ouwehand WH (1995) A human monoclonal antibody specific for the leucine 33 (P1A1, HPA 1a) form of platelet glycoprotein IIIa from a V gene phage display library. *Blood* **86**:4430–4436.

Griffiths AD, Malmqvist M, Marks JD, Bye JM, Embleton MJ, McCafferty J, Baier M, Holliger KP, Gorick BD, Hughes Jones NC, Winter G (1993) Human anti self antibodies with high specificity from phage display libraries. *EMBO J* **12**:725–734.

Griffiths AD, Williams SC, Hartley O, Tomlinson IM, Waterhouse P, Crosby WL, Kontermann RE, Jones PT, Low NM, Allison TJ (1994) Isolation of high affinity human antibodies directly from large synthetic repertoires. *EMBO J* **13**:3245–3260.

Grosjean H, Fiers W (1982) Preferential codon usage in prokaryotic genes: the optimal codon anticodon interaction energy and the selective codon usage in efficiently expressed genes. *Gene* **18**:199–209.

Hale G, Dyer MJ, Clark MR, Phillips JM, Marcus R, Ricchmann L, Winter G, Waldmann H (1988) Remission induction in non Hodgkin lymphoma with reshaped human monoclonal antibody CAMPATH 1H. *Lancet* **2**:1394–1399.

Hamers Casterman C, Atarhouch T, Muyldermans S, Robinson G, Hamers C, Songa EB, Bendahman N, Hamers R (1993) Naturally occurring antibodies devoid of light chains. *Nature* **363**:446–448.

Hawkins RE, Russell SJ, Winter G (1992) Selection of phage antibodies by binding affinity: minicking affinity maturation. *J Mol Biol* **226**:889–896.

Hayashi N, Welschof M, Zewe M, Braunagel M, Dübel S, Breitling F, Little M (1994) Simultaneous mutagenesis of antibody CDR regions by overlap extension and PCR. *Bio Techniques* **17**:310–313.

Hayden MS, Gilliland LK, Ledbetter JA (1997) Antibody engineering. *Curr Opin Immunol* **9**:201–212.

Hexham JM, Partridge LJ, Furmaniak J, Petersen VB, Colls JC, Pegg C, Rees Smith B, Burton DR (1994) Cloning and characterisation of TPO autoantibodies using combinatorial phage display libraries. *Autoimmunity* **17**:167–179.

Hirschmann R, Smith AB III, Taylor CM, Benkovic PA, Taylor SD, Yager KM, Sprengeler, POA, Benkovic SJ (1994) Peptide synthesis catalyzed by an antibody containing a binding site for variable amino acids. *Science* **265**:234–237.

Hollfelder F, Kirby AJ, Tawfik DS (1996) Off-the-shelf proteins that rival tailor-made antibodies as catalysts. *Nature* **383**:60–62.

Holz E, Raab R, Riethmuller G (1996) Antibody based immunotherapeutic strategies in colorectal cancer. *Recent Results Cancer Res* **142**:381–400.

Hoogenboom HR, Griffiths AD, Johnson KS, Chiswell DJ, Hudson P, Winter G (1991) Multi subunit proteins on the surface of filamentous phage: methodologies for displaying antibody (Fab) heavy and light chains. *Nucleic Acids Res* **19**:4133–4137.

Hughes-Jones NC, Gorick BD, Bye JM, Finnern R, Scott ML, Voak D, Marks JD, Ouwehand WH (1994) Characterization of human blood group scFv antibodies derived from a V gene phage display library. *Br J Haematol* **88**:180–186.

Huse WD, Sastry L, Iverson SA, Kang AS, Alting Mees M, Burton DR, Benkovic SJ, Lerner RA (1989) Generation of a large combinatorial library of the immunoglobulin repertoire in phage lambda. *Science* **246**:1275–1281.

Huston JS, Levinson D, Mudgett Hunter M, Tai MS, Novotny J, Margolies MN, Ridge RJ, Bruccolery RE, Haber E, Crea R, Oppermann H (1988) Protein engineering of antibody binding sites: recovery of specific activity in an anti digoxin single chain Fv analogue produced in *E. coli*. *Proc Natl Acad Sci USA* **85**:5879–5883.

Jacobsen JR, Schultz PG (1994) Antibody catalysis of peptide bond formation. *Proc Natl Acad Sci USA* **91**:6888–5892.

Jakobovits A (1995) Production of fully human antibodies by transgenic mice. *Curr Opin Biotechnol* **6**:561–566.

Janda KD, Lo CH, Li T, Barbas CF III, Wirsching P, Lerner RA (1994) Direct selection for a catalytic mechanism from combinatorial antibody libraries. *Proc Natl Acad Sci USA* **91**:2532–2536.

Jespers LS, Roberts A, Mahler SM, Winter G, Hoogenboom HR (1994) Guiding the selection of human antibodies from phage display repertoires to a single epitope of an antigen. *Biotechnology NY* **12**:899–903.

Jespers LS, Messens JH, De Keyser A, Eeckhout D, Van Den Brande I, Gansemans YG, Lauwereys MJ, Vlasuk GP, Stanssens PE (1995) Surface expression and ligand based selection of cDNAs fused to filamentous phage gene VI. *Bio/Technology* **13**:378–381.

Jung SH, Pastan I, Lee B (1994) Design of interchain disulfide bonds in the framework region of the Fv fragment of the monoclonal antibody B3. *Proteins* **19**:35–47.

Kabat EA, Wu TT, Reid Miller M, Perry HM, Gottesman KS (1987) Sequences of Proteins of Immunological Interest. U.S. Department of Health and Human Services, Public Health Service National Institutes of Health, Washington, DC.

Kang AS, Barbas CF, Janda KD, Benkovic SJ, Lerner RA (1991) Linkage of recognition and replication functions by assembling combinatorial antibody Fab libraries along phage surfaces. *Proc Natl Acad Sci USA* **88**:4363–4366.

Kirkpatrick RB, Ganguly S, Angelichio M, Griego S, Shatzman A, Silverman C, Rosenberg M (1995) Heavy chain dimers as well as complete antibodies are efficiently formed and secreted from *Drosophila* via a BIP mediated pathway. *J Biol Chem* **270**:19800–19805.

Krebber C, Spada S, Desplacq D, Plückthun A (1995) Coselection of cognate antibody antigen pairs by selectively infective phages. *FEBS Lett* **377**:227–231.

Lamers CH, Gratama JW, Warnaar SO, Stoter G, Bolhuis RL (1995) Inhibition of bispecific monoclonal antibody (bsAb) targeted cytolysis by human anti mouse antibodies in ovarian carcinoma patients treated with bsAb targeted activated T lymphocytes. *Int J Cancer* **60**:450–457.

Landry DW, Zhao K, Yang GX, Glickman M, Georgiadis TM (1993) Antibody catalyzed degradation of cocaine. *Science* **259**:1899–1901.

Lang IM, Barbas CF III, Schleef RR (1996) Recombinant rabbit Fab with binding activity to type 1 plasminogen activator inhibitor derived from a phage display library against human alpha granules. *Gene* **172**:295–298.

Lerner RA, Benkovic SJ, Schultz PG (1991) At the crossroads of chemistry and immunology: catalytic antibodies. *Science* **252**:659–667.

Lerner RA, Kang AS, Bain JD, Burton DR, Barbas CF III (1992) Antibodies without immunization. *Science* **258**:1313–1314.

Li L, Paul S, Tyutyulkova S, Kazatchkine MD, Kaveri S (1995) Catalytic activity of anti thyroglobulin antibodies. *J Immunol* **154**:3328–3332.

Lonberg N, Huszar D (1995) Human antibodies from transgenic mice. *Int Rev Immunol* **13**:65–93.

Low NM, Holliger P, Winter G (1996) Mimicking somatic hypermutation: affinity maturation of antibodies displayed on bacteriophage using a bacterial mutator strain. *J Mol Biol* **260**:359–368.

Lyttle MH, Napolitano EW, Calio BL, Kauvar LM (1995) Mutagenesis using trinucleotide beta cyanoethyl phosphoramidites. *Biotechniques* **19**:274–281.

Mallender WD, Carrero J, Voss EW Jr (1996) Comparative properties of the single chain antibody and Fv derivatives of mAb 4 4 20: relationship between interdomain interactions and high affinity for fluorescein ligand. *J Biol Chem* **271**:5338–5346.

Marks JD, Tristem M, Karpas A, Winter G (1991a) Oligonucleotide primers for polymerase chain reaction amplification of human immunoglobulin variable genes and design of family specific oligonucleotide probes. *Eur J Immunol* **21**:985–991.

Marks JD, Hoogenboom HR, Bonnert TP, McCafferty J, Griffiths AD, Winter G (1991b) By passing immunization: human antibodies from V gene libraries displayed on phage. *J Mol Biol* **222**:581–597.

Marks JD, Griffiths AD, Malmqvist M, Clackson TP, Bye JM, Winter G (1992) By passing immunization: building high affinity human antibodies by chain shuffling. *Biotechnology NY* **10**:779–783.

Marks JD, Ouwehand WH, Bye JM, Finnern R, Gorick BD, Voak D, Thorpe SJ, Hughes Jones NC, Winter G (1993) Human antibody fragments specific for human blood group antigens from a phage display library. *Bio/Technology* **11**:1145–1149.

Martin F, Toniatti C, Salvati AL, Venturini S, Ciliberto G, Cortese R, Sollazzo M (1994) The affinity selection of a minibody polypeptide inhibitor of human interleukin 6. *EMBO J* **13**:5305–5309.

McCafferty J, Griffiths AD, Winter G, Chiswel DJ (1990) Phage antibodies: filamentous phage displaying antibody variable domains. *Nature* **34**:552–554.

Merz DC, Dunn RJ, Drapeau P (1995) Generating a phage display antibody library against an identified neuron. *J Neurosc Methods* **62**:213–219.

Micheel B, Haymann S, Scharte G, Böttger V, Vogel F, Dübel S, Breitling F, Little M, Behrsing O (1994) Production of monoclonal antibodies against epitopes of the main coat protein of filamentous fd phages. *J Imm Methods* **171**:103–109.

Miyashita H, Karak Y, Kikuchi M, Fujii I (1993) Prodrug activation via catalytic antibodies. *Proc Natl Acad Sci USA* **90**:5337–5340.

Moosmayer D, Dübel S, Brocks B, Watzka H, Hampp C, Scheurich P, Little M, Pfizenmaler K (1995) A single chain TNF receptor antagonist is an effective inhibitor of TNF mediated cytotoxicity. *Ther Immunol* **2**:31–40.

Mullis K, Faloona F, Scharf S, Saiki R, Horn G, Erlich H (1992) Specific enzymatic amplification of DNA *in vitro*: the polymerase chain reaction. *Biotechnology* **24**:17–27.

Muyldermans S, Atarhouch T, Saldanha J, Barbosa JA, Hamers R (1994) Sequence and structure of VH domain from naturally occurring camel heavy chain immunoglobulins lacking light chains. *Protein Eng* **7**:1129–1135.

Nelson FK, Friedman SM, Smith GP (1981) Filamentous phage DNA cloning vectors: a non-infective mutant with a nonpolar deletion of gene III. *Virology* **108**:338–350.

Newton CR, Graham A (1994) PCR. Spektrum Akademischer Verlag, Heidelberg.

Nissim A, Hoogenboom HR, Tomlinson IM, Flynn G, Midgley C, Lane D, Winter G (1994) Antibody fragments from a 'single pot' phase display library as immunochemical reagents. *EMBO J* **13**:692–698.

Orlandi R, Güssow DH, Jones PT, Winter G (1989) Cloning immunoglobulin variable domains for expression by the polymerase chain reaction. *Proc Natl Acad Sci USA* **86**:3833–3837.

Ørum H, Andersen PS, Øster A, Johanse LK, Rüse E, Bjørnvad M, Svendsen I, Engberg J (1993) Efficient method for constructing comprehensive murine Fab antibody libraries displayed on phage. *Nucl Acid Res* **21**:4491–4498.

Pantoliano MW, Bird RE, Johnson S, Asel ED, Dodd SW, Wood JF, Hardman KD (1991) Conformational stability, folding and ligand binding affinity of single chain Fv immunoglobulin fragments expressed in *Escherichia coli*. *Biochemistry* **30**:10117–10125.

Parmley SF, Smith GP (1988) Antibody selectable filamentous fd phage vectors: affinity purification of target genes. *Gene* **73**:305–318.

Parren PW, Ditzel HJ, Gulizia RJ, Binley JM, Barbas CF III, Burton DR, Mosier DE (1995) Protection against HIV 1 infection in hu PBL SCID mice by passive immunization with a neutralizing human monoclonal antibody against gp120 CD4 binding site. *AIDS* **9**:1–6.

Paul S, Volle DJ, Beach CM, Johnson DR, Powell MJ, Massey RJ (1989) Catalytic hydrolysis of vasoactive intestinal peptide by human autoantibody. *Science* **243**:1158–1162.

Pessi A, Bianchi E, Crameri A, Venturini S, Tramontano A, Sollazzo MA (1993) Designed metal binding protein with a novel fold. *Nature* **362**:367–369.

Portolano S, McLachlan SM, Rapoport B (1993) High affinity, thyroid specific human autoantibodies displayed on the surface of filamentous phage use V genes similar to other autoantibodies. *J Immunol* **151**:2839–2851.

Powers JE, Machbank MT, Deutscher SL (1995) The isolation of U1 RNA binding antibody fragments from autoimmune human derived bacteriophage display libraries. *Nucleic Acids Symp Ser* **33**:240–243.

Raag R, Whitlow M (1995) Single chain Fvs. *FASEB J* **9**:73–80.

Rasched I, Oberer E (1986) Ff collphages: Structural and functional relationships, *Microbiol Rev* **50**:401–427.

Reiter Y, Brinkamann U, Kreitman RJ, Jung SH, Lee B, Pastan I (1994) Stabilization of the Fv fragments in recombinant immunotoxins by disulfide bonds engineered into conserved framework regions. *Biochemistry* **33**:5451–5459.

Reiter Y, Brinkamann U, Lee B, Pastan I (1996) Engineering antibody Fv-fragments for cancer detection and therapy: disulfide-stabilized Fv-fragments. *Nature Biotechnol* **14**:1239–1245.

Ridder R, Schmitz R, Legay F, Gram H (1995) Generation of rabbit monoclonal antibody fragments from a combinatorial phage display library and their production in the yeast *Pichia pastoris*. *Bio/Technology* **13**:255–260.

Riechmann L, Weill M (1993) Phage display and selection of a site directed randomized single chain antibody Fv fragment for its affinity improvement. *Biochemistry* **32**:8848–8855.

Riechmann L, Clark M, Waldmann H, Winter G (1988) Reshaping human antibodies for therapy. *Nature* **332**:323–327.

Riechmann L, Weill M, Cavanagh J (1992) Improving the antigen affinity of an antibody Fv fragment by protein design. *J Mol Biol* **224**:913–918.

Roberts VA, Stewart J, Benkovic SJ, Getzoff ED (1994) Catalytic antibody model and mutagenesis implicate arginine in transition state stabilization. *J Mol Biol* **235**:1098–1116.

Rondot S, Anthony K, Dübel S, Ida N, Beyreuther K, Frost L, Little M, Breitling F (1997) Epitopes fused to F Pilin are incorporated into functional recombinant pili. Submitted.

Rosenberg A, Griffin K, Studier EW, McCormick M, Berg J, Novy R, Mierendorf R (1996) T7Select Phage Display System: A powerful new protein display system based on bacteriophage 17. *in-Novations* **6**:2–7.

Russell SJ, Hawkins RE, Winter G (1993) Retroviral vectors displaying functional antibody fragments. *Nucleic Acids Res* **21**:1081–1085.

Sanna PP, Williamson RA, De Logu A, Bloom FE, Burton DR (1995) Directed selection of recombinant human monoclonal antibodies to herpes simplex virus glycoproteins from phage display libraries. *Proc Natl Acad Sci USA* **92**:6439–6445.

Sanna PP, De Logu A, Williamson RA, Hom YL, Straus SE, Bloom FE, Burton DR (1996) Protection of nude mice by passive immunization with a type common human recombinant monoclonal antibody against HSV. *Virology* **215**:101–106.

Saul FA, Poljak RJ (1993) Structural paterns at residue positions 9, 18, 67 and 82 in the VH framework regions of human and murine immunoglobulins. *J Mol Biol* **230**:15–20.

Schier R, Bye J, Apell G, McCall A, Adams GP, Malmqvist M, Weiner LM, Marks JD (1996) Isolation of high affinity monomeric human antic erbB 2 single chain Fv using affinity driven selection. *J Mol Biol* **255**:28–43.

Schiweck W, Skerra A (1997) The rational construction of an antibody against cystatin: lessons from the crystal structure of an artificial Fab fragment. *J Mol Biol* **269**:1–18.

Schnee JM, Runge MS, Matsueda GR, Hudson NW, Seidman JG, Haber E, Quertermous T (1987) Construction and expression of a recombinant antibody targeted plasminogen activator. *Proc Natl Acad Sci USA* **84**:6904–6908.

Schultz PG, Lerner RA (1995) From molecular diversity to catalysis: lessons from the immune system. *Science* **269**:1835–1842.

Scott JK, Smith GP (1990) Searching for peptide ligands with an epitope library. *Science* **249**:386–390.

Shuster AM, Gololobov GV, Kvashuk OA, Bogomolova AE, Smirnov IV, Gabibov AG (1992) DNA hydrolyzing autoantibodies. *Science* **256**:665–667.

Skerra A, Plückthun A (1988) Assembly of a functional immunoglobulin Fv fragment in *Escherichia coli*. *Science* **240**:1038–1041.

Skerra A, Dreher ML, Winter G (1991) Filter screening of antibody Fab fragments secreted from individual bacterial colonies: specific detection of antigen binding with a two membrane system. *Anal Biochem* **196**:151–155.

Smiley JA, Benkovic SJ (1994) Selection of catalytic antibodies for a biosynthetic reaction from a combinatorial cDNA library by complementation of an auxotrophic *Escherichia coli*: antibodies for orotate decarboxylation. *Proc Natl Acad Sci USA* **91**:8319–8323.

Smith GP (1985) Filamentous fusion phage: novel expression vectors that display cloned antigens on the virion surface. *Science* **228**:1315–1317.

Soderlind E, Vergeles M, Borrebaeck CA (1995) Domain libraries: syntheric diversity for *de novo* design of antibody V regions. *Gene* **160**:269–272.

Sondek J, Shortle DA (1992) General strategy for random insertion and substitution mutagenesis: substoichiometric coupling of trinucleotide phosphoramidites. *Proc Natl Acad Sci USA* **89**:3581–3585.

Song Z, Cai Y, Song D, Xu J, Yuan H, Wang L, Zhu X, Lin H, Breitling F, Dübel S (1997) Primary structure and functional expression of heavy- and light-chain variable region genes of a monoclonal antibody specific for human fibrin. *Hybridoma* **16**:235–241.

Songsivila S, Bye JM, Marks JD, Hughes Jones NC (1990) Cloning and sequencing of human lambda immunoglobulin genes by the polymerase chain reaction. *Eur J Immunol* **20**:2661–2666.

Soumillion P, Jespers L, Bouchet M, Marchand Brynaert J, Winter G, Fastrez J (1994) Selection of beta lactamase of filamentous bacteriophage by catalytic activity. *J Mol Biol* **237**:415–422.

Spinelli S, Frenken L, Bourgeols D, deRou L, Bos W, Verrips T, Anquille C, Cambillan C, Tegoni M (1996) The crystal structure of allame heavy chain variable domain. *Nat Struct Biol* **3**:752–757.

Stemmer WP (1994) Rapid evolution of a protein *in vitro* by DNA shuffling. *Nature* **370**:389–391.

Stemmer WP, Morris SK, Wilson BS (1993) Selection of an active single chain Fv antibody from a protein linker library prepared by enzymatic inverse PCR. *Biotechniques* **14**:256–265.

Stryhn A, Andersen PS, Pedersen LO, Svejgaard A, Holm A, Thorpe CJ, Fugger L, Buus S, Engberg J (1996) Shared fine specifity between T-cell receptors and an antibody recognizing a peptide/major histocompatibility class I complex. *Proc Natl Acad Sci USA* Vol **93**:10338–10342.

Studnicka GM, Soares S, Better M, Williams RE, Nadell R, Horwitz AH (1994) Human engineered monoclonal antibodies retain full specific binding activity by preserving non CDR complementarity modulating residues. *Protein Eng* **7**:805–814.

Süsal C, Groth J, Oberg HH, Ternes P, May G, Opelz G (1992) The association of kidney graft outcome with pretransplant serum IgG anti F (ab')2 gamma activity. *Transplantation* **54**:632–635.

Takkinen K, Laukkanen ML, Sizmann D, Alfthan K, Immonen T, Vanne L, Kaartinen M, Knowles JK, Teeri TT (1991) An active single chain antibody containing a cellulase linker domain is secreted by *Escherichia coli. Protein Eng* **4**:837–841.

Tang Y, Hicks JB, Hilvert D (1991) *In vivo* catalysis of a metabolically essential reaction by an antibody. *Proc Natl Acad Sci USA* **88**:8784–8786.

Tang Y, Jiang N, Parakh C, Hilvert D (1996) Selection of linkers for a catalytic single chain antibody using phage display technology. *J Biol Chem* **271**:15682–15686.

Terness P, Kirschfink M, Navolan D, Dufter C, Kohl I, Opelz G, Roelcke D (1995) Striking inverse correlation between IgG anti F(ab')2 and autoantibody production in patients with cold agglutination. *Blood* **85**:548–551.

Tomlinson IM, Cox JP, Gherardi E, Lesk AM, Chothia C (1995) The structural repertoire of the human V kappa domain. *EMBO J* **14**:548–551.

Tramontano A, Chothia C, Lesk AM (1990) Framework residue 71 is a major determinant of the position and conformation of second hypervariable region in the VH domains of immunoglobulins. *J Mol Biol* **215**:175–182.

Tsunenari T, Akamatsu K, Kaiho S, Sato K, Tsuchiya M, Koishihara Y, Kishimoto T, Ohsugi Y (1996) Therapeutic potential of humanized anti interleukin 6 receptor antibody: antitumor activity in xenograft model of multiple myeloma. Anticancer Res **16**:2537–2544.

Tsurushita N, Fu H, Warren C (1996) Phage display vectors for *in vivo* recombination of immunoglobulin heavy and light chain genes to make large combinatorial libraries. *Gene* **172**:59–63.

Utsumi S, Karush F (1964) Subunits of purified rabbit antibody. *Biochemistry* **3**:1329–1338.

Vargas-Madrazo E, Lara Ochoa F, Almagro JC (1995) Canonical structure repartoire of the antigen binding site of immunoglobulins suggests strong geometrical restriction associated to the mechanism of immune recognition. *J Mol Biol* **254**:497–504.

Virnekas B, Ge L, Plückthun A, Schneider KC, Wellnhofer G, Moroney SE (1994) Trinucleotide phosphoramidites: ideal reagents for the synthesis of mixed oligonucleotides for random mutagenesis. *Nucleic Acids Res* **22**:5600–5607.

Ward ES, Gussow D, Griffiths AD, Jones PT, Winter G (1989) Binding activities of a repertoire of single immunoglobulin variable domains secreted from *Escherichia coli. Nature* **341**:544–546.

Ward VK, Kreissig SB, Hammock BD, Choudary PV (1996) Generation of an expression library in the baculovirus expression vector system. *J Virol Methods* **53**:263–272.

Webster RE, Lopez J (1985) Structure and assembly of the class 1 filamentous bacteriophage. Casjens S, editor. Virus Structure and Assembly. Jones and Bartlett, Boston pp 235–267.

Welschof M, Terness P, Kolbinger F, Zewe M, Dübel S, Dörsam H, Hain C, Finger M, Jung M, Moldenhauer G, Hayashi N, Little M, Opelz G (1995) Amino acid sequence based PCR primers for amplification of rearranged human heavy and light chain immunoglobulin variable region genes. *J Immunol Methods* **179**:203–214.

Welschof M, Terness P, Kipriyanov S, Stanescu, Breitling F, Dorsam H, Dübel S, Little M, Opelz G (1997a) the antigen binding domain of a human IgG anti F(ab')2 autoantibody. *Proc Natl Acad Sci USA* **94**:1902–1907.

Welschof M, Little M, Dörsam H (1997b) Production of a human antibody library in the phage-display vector pSEX81. Methods Mol Med.

Wentworth P, Datta A, Blakey D, Boyle T, Partridge LJ, Blackburn GM (1996) Toward antibody directed "abzyme" prodrug therapy ADAPT: carbamate prodrug activation by a catalytic antibody and its *in vitro* application to human tumor cell killing. *Proc Natl Acad Sci USA* **93**:799–803.

Williams MN, Freshour G, Darvill AG, Albershein P, Hahn MG (1996) An antibody Fab selected from a recombinant phage display library detects deesterified pectic polysaccharide rhamnogalacturonan II in plant cells. *Plant Cell* **8**:673–685.

Williamson RA, Burioni R, Sanna PP, Partridge LJ, Barbas CF III, Burton DR (1993) Human monoclonal antibodies against a plethora of viral pathogens from single combinatorial libraries. *Proc Natl Acad Sci USA* **90**:4141–4145.

Winter G, Harris WJ (1993) Humanized antibodies. *Immunol Today* **14**:243–246.

Winter G, Griffiths AD, Hawkins RE, Hoogenboom HR (1994) Making antibodies by phage display technology. *Annu Rev Immunol* **12**:433–455.

Wirsching P, Ashley JA, Lo CH, Janda KD, Lerner RA (1995) Reactive immunization. *Science* **270**:1775–1782.

Wright A, Shin SU, Marrison SL (1992) Genetically engineered antibodies: progress and prospects. *Crit Rev immunol* **12**:125–168.

Yamanaka HI, Inoue T, Ikeda Tanaka O (1996) Chicken monoclonal antibody isolated by a phage display system. *Immunol* **157**:1156–1162.

Yang WP, Green K, Pinz Sweeney S, Briones AT, Burton DR, Barbas CF III (1995) CDR walking mutagenesis for the affinity maturation of a potent human anti HIV 1 antibody into the picomolar range. *J Mol Biol* **254**:392–403.

Zebedee SL, Barbas CF III, Hom YL, Caothien RH, Gaff R, DeGraw J, Pyati J, LaPolla R, Burton DR, Lerner RA (1992) Human combinational antibody libraries to hepatitis B surface antigen. *Proc Natl Acad Sci USA* **89**:3175–3179.

Zhou GW, Guo J, Huang W, Fletterick RJ, Scanlan TS (1994) Crystal structure of a catalytic antibody with a serine protease active site. *Science* **265**:1059–1064.

Ziegler A, Torrance L, Macintosh SM, Cowan GH, Mayo MA (1995) Cucumber mosaic cucumovirus antibodies from a synthetic phage display library. *Virology* **214**:235–238.

Chapter 3
Antibodies With New Functions

3.1 Why Bispecific and Bifunctional Antibodies?

Polyclonal and monoclonal antibodies have long been proven to be valuable tools in diagnosis. Due to their high specificity, a diversity of diseases and infections can be diagnosed with their help. The first HIV tests, for example, were based on the binding of monoclonal antibodies to the viral antigen. There is, however, no comparable success story for antibodies in the treatment of diseases, although they should be ideal therapeutic tools in many diseases because of their extraordinary ability to make distinctions. In part, this is surely because only in a few cases, binding to antigen alone is sufficient to achieve a therapeutic effect. Examples of such exceptions include an antibody fragment against tumor necrosis factor (Orfanoudakis et al., 1993) or its receptor (Moosmayer et al., 1995), which can function as an antagonist of signal transduction and thus, may limit potentially life-threatening inflammatory reactions. An antibody against myelin-associated neurite growth inhibitor stimulates nerve regeneration by neutralizing the inhibitor (Bandtlow et al., 1996). An scFv antibody against the antidepressive drug, desipramine, can be used to neutralize the circulating drug (Shelver et al., 1996). The large amount of antibody fragments needed for such neutralization applications, however, can become a problem (Keyler et al., 1994). Most therapeutic applications therefore use modified antibodies, in which the antibody domains provide only the binding specificity, whereas the therapeutic effect is mediated by an additional effector.

In particular, tumor-specific antibodies (see Section 2.3.6.3) could become very valuable, if a toxic element could be selectively targeted to the tumor. The better the antibody can distinguish the normal tissue from the closely related tumor, the less the damage to the healthy tissue. This, again, means that the cancer can be more efficiently fought because more of the therapeutic agent reaches the tumor. Therefore, the chances of a cure increase (Bodey et al., 1996).

Recombinant antibody technology first enabled the production of a new quality as well as larger quantities of human antibodies (see also Section 2.3.6). Correspondingly, almost without exception, antibodies from mice were used until now for cancer therapy, with all the drawbacks that the use of these foreign proteins in humans brings (see also Section 2.4.2 and Fig. 2.14). This is certainly one of the most important reasons for the frequent failure of antibody therapy. There is probably another, deeper-lying reason for this, however. Many tumors apparently initiate a distinct and specific immune response, during which the cancer patient forms antibodies against tumor-associated antigens (Sahin et al., 1995). The tumor, however continues to grow in these patients. These antibodies are obviously not able to fight the tumor successfully alone. The reason for this could be that, apart from antigen binding, further signals are necessary for the successful destruction of the tumor. A cytotoxic T-cell, for instance, requires at least two signals before it destroys a target cell. The first, specific signal is the recognition of the antigen by the T-cell receptor, but the cytotoxic T-cell is only activated when it simultaneously binds a costimulatory molecule, such as CD28 of the target cell (see overview in Janeway and Travers, 1997). This "backup insurance" of the immune system makes sense because, otherwise, the damage by for example, cross-reactions with self-antigens that single B- or T-cell clones could cause could not be limited.

This is the main reason why great hope is placed on therapy with the help of recombinant antibodies that can be altered with relative ease, using molecular biological techniques. Modern methods of gene technology can combine completely different molecules with each other, from which the antibody can gain almost any additional properties (Fig. 3.1). This enables the necessary additional signals to be connected to the recombinant antibody fragment, often with the hope that, in this way, the immune system can be specifically activated against a tumor cell (Fig. 3.2) (Bohlen et al., 1993b; Hartmann et al., 1996).

The previous chapters were concerned with the properties of the antigen binding site: binding specificity, affinity, size, and stability. The following sections focus on the predominantly medical applications of these fragments, that is, the binding specificity of the antibody fragment should be exploited to mark or destroy the target, to encapsulate it, to impede it, or to change it.

An antibody rarely functions solely based on its binding to antigen. Therefore, the normal antibodies formed by our immune system also have at

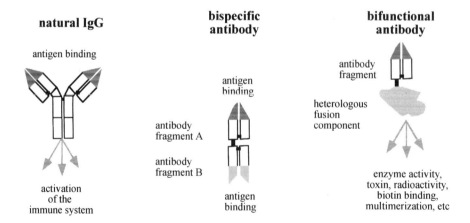

Fig. 3.1. Natural immunoglobulins can of course be considered to be bifunctional antibodies because they not only bind antigen but also mediate further functions, such as complement activation. The term *bifunctional antibody*, however, has come in to use for artificially produced constructs. *Bispecific* antibodies can bind to two different antigens. *Bifunctional* antibodies possess activities that natural immunoglobulins do not provide.

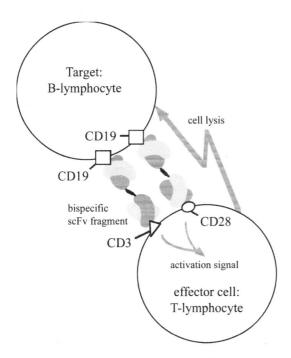

Fig. 3.2. Bispecific antibodies mobilize the T-lymphocyte defense. Example: a B-cell lymphoma expresses the differentiation antigen CD19. A bispecific antibody guides the cytotoxic activity of a T-cell to the target cell by the combination of anti-CD19-anti-CD3 and anti-CD19-anti-CD28 antibodies.

least two functions (*bifunctional*). One function is the specific recognition of the antigen, which has been described in Chapter 2. The second function, however, activates the immune system. The constant domains of our antibodies call to the immune system for help. Different constant areas activate different subsystems of the immune system (Table 3.1).

Table 3.1   Structure and Effector Functions of the Immunoglobulin Classes

Class	Heavy Chain	Antigen-Binding Sites	Function Location	Functions
IgM	μ	10	Bloodstream	Primary immune response; complement activation, agglutination
IgG	γ	2	Bloodstream	Secondary immune response; complement activation, neutralization, opsonization
IgA	α	2, 4, or 6	Secretions, breast milk	Neutralization at the body surface, intestinal immunity of newborns
IgE	ε	2	Subcutaneous, submucosal	Sensitization of mast cells, activation of eosinophils
IgD	δ	2	Surface of B cells	Receptor for the stimulation of the B cell through the antigen

The recombinant antibody fragment usually performs the specific recognition of the target, and the fusion partner performs the desired second function. A few examples follow that will be discussed later in detail. The fusion partner can be a second, different antibody fragment. Such *bispecific* constructs can enable a T-lymphocyte, for example, to lyse tumor cells (Fig. 3.2). Heterologous fusion partners, that is, those from other organisms or with other tasks, can also be fused with recombinant antibody fragments into *bifunctional* antibodies. Fusion with a toxin yields a specifically binding cytotoxin (immunotoxin). A radioactive atom as a binding partner reveals the exact location of a tumor and its metastases by its decay, detectable by immunoscintigraphy. An enzyme can also be transported to the tumor site through an antibody fragment. A nontoxic precursor substance can then be transformed into a toxic substance and thus, kill adjacent tumor cells as well. Recombinant antibodies can even be expressed within cells and thus protect cells from viruses such as HIV.

3.2 New Functions Through Homologous Fusion Partners: Bispecific Antibodies

3.2.1 BISPECIFIC ANTIBODIES UNITE THE BINDING PROPERTIES OF TWO DIFFERENT MONOCLONAL ANTIBODIES INTO ONE MOLECULE

With the introduction of hybridoma technology by Köhler and Milstein in 1975, molecules became available that could bind with high selectivity to target molecules. If two of these monoclonal antibodies are now joined by chemical coupling or by the fusion of two hybridoma cells, a *bispecific* antibody is formed. These hybrid molecules unite the binding properties of two different monoclonal antibodies into one molecule. They are artificial molecules that do not occur in nature.

More than thirty years ago, bispecific $F(ab')_2$ fragments were produced by the oxidation of monovalent F(ab') fragments (Nisonoff and Rivers, 1961). Bispecific antibodies can also be directly synthesized from cells. In 1983, Milstein and Cuello (1983) fused two different hybridoma cells with each other for the first time. One hybridoma cell secreted an antiperoxidase antibody, the other an antisomatostatin antibody. The resulting *hybrid hybridoma* (or *quadroma*) cell produced the desired bispecific antibody, and additionally, nine other variants that had to be separated from the desired bispecific molecule (Fig. 3.3). This is often difficult because the different molecules are usually very similar to one another so that often only an affinity purification with both immobilized antigens yields the desired product. Therefore, the production of

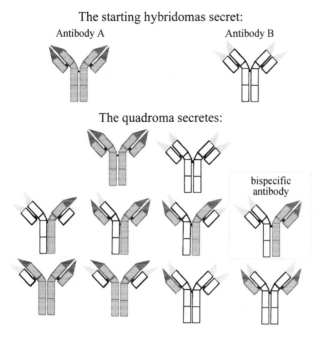

Fig. 3.3. Given that no preference occurs in the chain pairing, the quadroma (hybrid hybridoma) cells secrete *10* different IgG variants. Only *1* of these variants is the desired bispecific antibody.

bispecific antibodies from quadromas is enormously expensive. However, the advantages of this method still outweighed that of the chemical coupling of two antibodies because the position and stoichiometry of the coupling are fixed, and there is no danger that the areas important for antigen binding in the hyper-variable regions are inactivated through covalent modification.

Why is there now such great interest in these molecules?

3.2.1.1 Bispecific Antibodies Can Selectively Join Different Cells or Molecules

Bispecific antibodies can highly specifically join two partners, cells, or molecules with each other. Thus, the possibility exists, for example, to intervene in the disrupted communication between tumor cells and the immune system. Some tumors are apparently tolerated by the immune system, although they possess tumor-associated antigens, against which patients have antibodies (Sahin et al., 1995). Meanwhile, in many model systems, this tolerance to the tumors has been successfully overcome by using bispecific antibodies. A tumor-specific antibody is joined with one or several antibodies that activate the immune system. Potential target structures are surface molecules, such as CD2, CD3, and CD28 on T-cells or CD16 on NK cells. Macrophages can also be activated by binding to CD64 (Fanger et al., 1994; Fanger, 1995; Demanet et al., 1996; Hartmann et al., 1996).

The recombinant techniques of molecular biology allows a modular composition. A tumor-specific antibody can also be joined with other partners, for example, with an antibody that recognizes a radioactive hapten (Lollo et al., 1994). Similarly, the "target seeking head" can be exchanged so that a functional effector system can be conducted to different tumors with the help of various antibodies.

In a further application, the receptor-mediated endocytosis is exploited to transport a toxic cargo inside tumor cells. Here, one arm of the bispecific antibody binds to the receptor while the other binds the cargo, which is transported inside the cells through the internalizing receptor. One of many examples is the transport of saporin into the cell interior of neoplastic T-cells. In this case, the receptor was the T-cell antigen CD25. Saporin concentrations of less than 10^{-11} mol/l were sufficient for a 50% inactivation of the ribosomes (Tazzari et al., 1993).

Besides this, there is an abundance of other applications for bispecific antibodies (Fanger, 1995). For example, the maturation of T-cells can be examined with their help. T-cells are seemingly altered by contact with certain cells in the thymus. Bispecific antibodies are an elegant aid in the investigation into which contacts are important and in what order they occur (Müller and Kyewski, 1995).

3.2.1.2 Tumors Can Be Better Detected With Bispecific Antibodies

The fundamental problem in the diagnosis of tumors is the same as that for treatment: the tumor must be recognized as specifically as possible. Antibodies are potentially very suitable for this task due to their high specificity. Today, sufficient specific antibodies are available for various tumor diagnoses. A problem that has been addressed many times must be solved. The antibody must be able to diffuse into the tumor interior. This diffusion needs time. A high concentration of the tumor-specific antibody must be maintained in the patient's bloodstream for several days if possible, so that enough antibody can diffuse into the tumor body, and anchor there through its specific binding. This can lead to severe, intolerable side-effects for the patient if the antibody is loaded with a radioactive nuclide (for diagnosis) or even with a toxin (for therapy) for this entire, lengthy time span.

This problem can be handled with a trick. First, the patient is given a high concentration of the tumor specific antibody over a long period. The antibody, which is harmless to the patient, concentrates in the tumors. When a bispecific antibody is used for this, a second binding specificity is available that can be directed against a small hapten. This hapten can now be coupled to a toxin or a radioactive nuclide. The resulting molecule can be very small and this diffuse into the tumor very quickly. In tumor diagnosis, the hapten is bound to a short-lived radioactive nuclide and concentrates in the tumor in a few hours or even minutes. Unbound hapten (and the radioactivity) is quickly excreted through the kidneys. The radioactive marker discloses the exact position of the tumor and its metastases in immunoscintigraphy. Thus, the patient is subjected to the radioactivity for a short time (Peltier et al., 1993; Somasundaram et al., 1993; Schumacher et al., 1995). The size of the antibody can also dramatically influence its pharmacological properties. This is detailed in Section 4.2.1.2.

3.2.1.3 Bispecific Antibodies Can Combat Tumor Cells

Bispecific antibodies have already proved their ability to kill tumor cells in many cell culture systems selectively (Bohlen et al., 1993a; Kurucz et al., 1995; Zhu et al., 1995). One arm of the bispecific antibody is assigned to specific tumor recognition (Bohlen et al., 1993b; Link and Weiner, 1993; Holliger et al., 1996).

The effector functions are mediated by the second arm, for which two different approaches are currently favored. The effector molecule can be a cancer toxin that is externally administered. This is described more thoroughly in Chapter 3.3. An effector molecule that activates the patient's immune system can also be used, through which it destroys cells marked by the bispecific antibody. A practicable option is the activation of cytotoxic T-lymphocytes by an anti-CD3 antibody in combination with an anti-CD28 antibody (Bohlen et al., 1993a) (see Fig. 3.2). *Natural killer* cells, granulocytes, and macrophages can also be activated through CD16 with another effector arm (Kurucz et al., 1995; Segal et al., 1995; Ely et al., 1996). These *in vitro* experiments could be an important milestone on the road to a selective tumor therapy that perhaps, one day, may spare the patient from the relatively unspecific effects of chemo- or radiotherapy (Holliger and Winter, 1993; Bodey et al., 1996).

Animal models already exist for several bispecific antibodies (Bakacs et al., 1995; Weiner et al., 1995a). In a particularly impressive example, a Hodgkin lymphoma was successfully combated with bispecific antibodies. In this instance, an antibody directed against the surface molecule CD30 on the tumor cells of the Hodgkin lymphoma served as the tumor-specific arm. A bispecific anti-CD30, anti-CD3 antibody could not protect the mice from the tumors alone. In combination with a bispecific anti-CD30, anti-CD28 antibody however, the tumor was completely destroyed (Hartmann et al., 1996).

There are now the first therapeutic attempts in human tumor patients using bispecific antibodies of murine origin, most of which are produced by hybrid hybridomas. Still only a few patients can be treated in this way because the production and purification of these bispecific antibodies are currently extremely cost- and labor-intensive. In most of the patients treated, the incidence of side-effects was low; however, the majority developed a strong immune response against the administered mouse immunoglobulin (HAMA) (Lamers et al., 1995; Weiner et al., 1995b). The possibility exists to overcome this problem with recombinant, bispecific Fv fragments produced in *E. coli*. Such constructs will probably soon reach the stage of clinical trials.

3.2.2 RECOMBINANT PRODUCTION OF BISPECIFIC ANTIBODIES

As described in the previous chapters, Fv or Fab fragments can be produced in *E. coli* using recombinant DNA techniques. In contrast to the hybridoma cells, antibody genes can easily be modified and combined in *E. coli*. A recombinant production of bispecific antibodies therefore avoids the drawbacks of by products in quadromas (Fig. 3.3), and the ambiguity of chemical

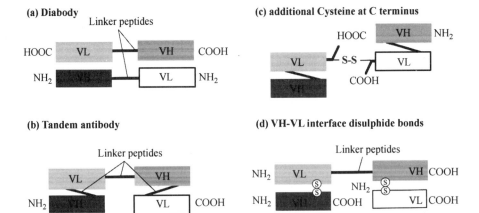

Fig. 3.4. Options for producing recombinant bispecific antibodies. (**a**) Diabodies (not covalently coupled). (**b**) Tandem antibody. (**c**) Through oxidation of C terminal cysteines. (**d**) Through disulfide bridges at the VH–VL interface.

coupling. Additionally, a bispecific antibody formed in *E. coli* can be produced in large quantities (reviewed in Carter et al., 1995). Several ways to generate bispecific antibodies in *E. coli* are shown below (Fig. 3.4).

3.2.2.1 Bispecific Diabodies Result When Two scFv Fragments Are Expressed Inside The Same Cell

In the purification of scFv fragments expressed in *E. coli* over a gel filtration column, a considerable portion of these scFv fragments clearly formed dimers. The quantity of dimers depends on the length of the peptide link between the two variable domains. The shorter the linker the more dimers are formed (Raag and Whitlow, 1995). X-ray crystallography shows that each pair of scFv fragments lie head to tail. The VH domain of one scFv fragment pairs with the VL domain of the other. This yielded the blueprint for the design of a bispecific diabody. The expression cassettes for two different scFv fragments are needed, whose variable domains have been exchanged, that is, one scFv fragment expresses the VH domain of Fv fragment A followed by the VL domain of Fv fragment B. In the other scFv fragment it is reversed: VH(B) is followed by VL(A) (Holliger et al., 1993; Perisic et al., 1994). Meanwhile, there are even diabody gene libraries, from which bispecific diabodies may be directly selected. The genes for the diabody are linked with the phage coat protein pIII, similar to that described for scFv fragments in Section 2.3.5 (McGuinness et al., 1996).

Bispecific antibodies need not be used merely to connect two different molecules. When they recognize two adjacent epitopes on the same molecule or cell, they bind more specifically compared with the monospecific antibodies. This is of interest when only two, poor quality, monospecific antibodies are available for a tumor cell. The publication from Hakalahti and colleagues (1993) shows that a bispecific antibody thus obtained, can, indeed, increase the binding specificity for tumor cells. This was also true for a bispecific recombinant diabody (Fig. 3.4a), whose two binding arms recognized two different epitopes on the enzyme lysozyme. Compared with the monospecific scFv fragments, a more than 10-fold increased affinity for the antigen was detected with these so-called CRABS (Neri et al., 1995a).

The stability of diabodies however, is not very high and this can cause problems. Dimers could form tetramers and so forth. Insoluble aggregates and nonspecific binding can result from high protein concentrations. There is also no guarantee that only the desired heterodimers will be formed. Moreover, two heterodimers can rearrange into two homodimers in solution and reversed. The rate of this rearrangement depends on the (often low) binding constants of the variable domains for each other. Most of these criticisms apply not only to the formation of diabodies, but also always when scFv fragments are used in the construction of a bispecific antibody (Raag and Whitlow, 1995). For diabodies, however, the binding energy of the domains additionally supplies the coupling energy for the fragments.

3.2.2.2 Tandem Antibodies

A direct method for producing bispecific antibodies is the tandem fusion of two scFv fragments (Fig. 3.4b). Here, the genes of both scFv fragments are joined with a peptide linker so that all four variable regions lie one after the other in a single peptide strand. When expressed in *E. coli*, this leads to bispecific antibodies that have to be renatured however, and are obtained only in small yields (Carter et al., 1995; Kranz et al., 1995).

3.2.2.3 Bispecific Antibodies Can Be Produced by the Oxidation of Two scFv Fragments

Natural immunoglobulins are stabilized through disulfide bridges. Each domain forms an *intra*molecular disulfide bridge, whereas the chains participating in the construction of an antibody molecule are connected through *inter*molecular disulfide bridges (see Fig. 1.1). An additional disulfide bridge can be formed with recombinant techniques, which opens up the possibility of connecting two scFv fragments by oxidation. The scFv fragments can be individually purified and then connected, *in vitro*, with the help of the C-terminal cysteines (Fig. 3.4c) (Cumber et al., 1992; Kipriyanov et al., 1994). In addition, this trick can be combined with the use of a dimerization domain (see below) (de Kruif and Logtenberg, 1996).

3.2.2.4 Disulfide Bridges at the VH–VL Interface Can Be Used in the Construction of Bispecific Antibodies

Bispecific antibodies should be as small as possible in the treatment of solid tumors, so that they can better enter the malignant tissue. Among others, scFv fragments fulfill this criterion at best, and are therefore an obvious choice, for use as building blocks in the construction of bispecific antibodies. scFv fragments however, often do not have the desired stability (see also Section 2.4.1).

The insertion of an additional intramolecular disulfide bridge (see Section 2.4.10) at the VH-VL *interface* can help, resulting in so-called dsFv fragments.

Two different places can be used for the stabilization through a disulfide bridge of two scFv fragments of different specificities. This can be exploited for the construction of bispecific antibodies (Fig. 3.4d). Both dsFv fragments are formed in the same cell. A disulfide bridge can only form when the cysteines involved fit exactly to one another (Little et al., 1994) (Breitling and Dübel, unpublished observations). Because of their low affinity, both variable domains will dissociate if a covalent coupling through a disulfide bridge does not occur. This selects for the connection of the correct VH and VL domains. Only one peptide link is required between the two variable domains of both fragments with different specificities to construct the bispecific antibodies.

3.2.3 CREATING BISPECIFIC ANTIBODIES WITH HELP FROM HETEROLOGOUS BINDING DOMAINS

For several years, protein domains called "leucine zippers" have been known from research on transcription factors. An ordered sequence of leucines causes a dimerization of these short, C-terminal peptides. The leucine zippers of the transcription factors *fos* and *jun* are of particular interest. The formation of *jun/fos* heterodimers is preferred to the respective homodimers when the two structures are added together (Alberts et al., 1994). The fusion of antibody fragments to both of these domains does not change this. The majority of the molecules formed were heterodimers, that is, antibody fragments with two different specificities (Fig. 3.5a). Similar to the fusion of two hybridoma cells, the desired bispecific antibody must first be separated from the homodimers. The proportion of desired bispecific antibodies, however, is clearly greater (Kostelny et al., 1992; Pack et al., 1993). Following the same principle, Fv fragments with four binding valencies were produced with the help of the tetramerization domain of the p53 molecule (Rheinnecker et al., 1996).

The fusion of an antibody fragment to the small protein calmodulin can also be employed (Fig. 3.5b). In the presence of calcium ions, calmodulin binds to peptides such as mastoparan with very high affinity (up to 3×10^{-10} mol/l). When the calcium ions are complexed with EGTA, the binding is dissolved. This enables a very gentle affinity purification of the antibody fragment. When a second antibody is chemically or genetically fused to a calmodulin binding peptide, the mixture yields bispecific antibodies. In this method, all the resulting molecules should, theoretically, be able to participate in the construction of bispecific antibodies, because homodimers do not arise (Neri et al., 1995b). Calmodulin is a human protein that is only weakly immunogenic. Therefore, the danger is minimal that it results in difficulties, analogous to the HAMA, when used in patients (see also, Section 2.4.2).

A further possibility is the fusion of a recombinant antibody fragment to protein A from *Staphylococcus aureus*. Protein A (see also Section 4.4.3.3) recognizes the constant areas of many antibodies, so that this recombinant fusion protein can be combined with existing hybridoma antibodies to form a diversity of bispecific antibodies (Fig. 3.5c). In one example, an anti-CD3 scFv

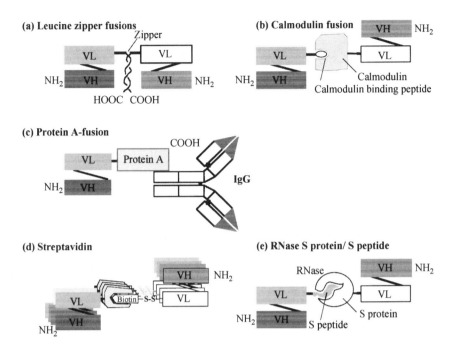

Fig. 3.5. Production of recombinant bispecific antibodies by the use of heterologous dimerization domains. (**a**) With the help of a leucine zipper. (**b**) Through fusion to calmodulin or a calmodulin binding peptide. (**c**) Through fusion to a fragment of protein A. (**d**) Through fusion to streptavidin (with a biotinylated partner). (**e**) Through fusion to two different fragments of an RNase.

fragment was fused to protein A. The anti-CD3 portion can activate cytotoxic T-cells, which can then destroy those cells recognized by the second antibody partner. Thus, a quick test is at hand with which to search for suitable candidates for tumor-specific, bispecific antibodies. A disadvantage of this method is that protein A is recognized as foreign by the human immune system and, therefore, hardly any intensive therapeutic use is possible. Additionally, such bispecific antibodies are not stable in the bloodstream because antibodies from the serum also compete for binding to the protein A.

3.2.3.1 Bispecific Antibodies Acquire an Additional Enzymatic Property Through the Fusion to RNase S Peptide and S Protein

Similarly, bispecific antibodies can be produced when the antibody fragments are fused to two enzyme fragments that can reform the complete enzyme. This, for example, is possible for human ribonuclease A. The enzyme fragments, S protein and S peptide, are fused to different scFv fragments (Fig. 3.5e). Bispecific antibodies with RNase activity result upon mixing (Dübel, 1999). This RNase activity may be of use, for example, as a bispecific immunotoxin, for the specific destruction of tumor cells (see Section 3.3.2.4). An advantage is not only the stoichiometrically correct and defined pairing of both scFv fragments. The binding affinity can also be greatly increased, compared with that for common immunotoxins, by combination with different tumor-marker antibodies (see Section 3.2.2.1). As with all immunotoxins, however, this construct must reach the inside of cells, that is, at least one of the scFv fragments must be directed against an internalizing antigen.

3.2.4 "UNIVERSAL" BISPECIFIC ANTIBODIES

Although the expression of antibody fragments in *E. coli* has considerably simplified the construction and modification of bispecific antibodies, the construction of a new bispecific antibody is still very labor-intensive. This was the incentive for the construction of the *universal bispecific antibodies*. These were not constructed for a narrowly confined purpose, but to allow a wide range of applications. The universal use is enabled through a fusion protein that can bind two different haptens. This fragment can now combine nearly every desired partner to another, as long as these were previously coupled to the haptens. An example of such a universal antibody fragment is the fusion of a scFv fragment to streptavidin (Dübel et al., 1995), in which the scFv fragment recognizes a short peptide epitope, a small hapten or the constant parts of immunoglobulin chains (Dübel and Breitling, unpublished observations). The other partner either is coupled to biotin chemically, or it can be already biotinylated *in vivo* by fusion to the *E. coli* protein BCCP, as shown for a Fab' fragment against TNF (Weiss et al., 1994).

This approach, of course, can be limited to one binding arm. When, for example, one is bound to a hapten, that is, a universal scFv fragment bound to a tumor-specific antibody fragment, the radioactively marked hapten can be used to mark the tumor (Lollo et al., 1994). It can also be coupled to an existing monoclonal antibody that activates the immune system against the tumor (George et al., 1994). In another example, this application enabled an antibody-mediated infection of target cells. The hapten (this time a small peptide epitope) is expressed on the surface of a recombinant adenovirus. The universal portion of the bispecific antibody fragment binds the target cell with one arm while the other recognizes the peptide epitope and therefore the recombinant virus (Wickham et al., 1996).

3.2.5 RECOMBINANT BISPECIFIC ANTIBODIES CAN BE DISTINCTLY SMALLER THAN AN IgG

A bispecific antibody composed of two Fv fragments (e.g., a diabody) is about as large as a Fab fragment and is therefore about one-third the size of an IgG of around 160 kDa. For many applications, this size difference is a decided advantage. This property is especially interesting in the prospective treatment of tumors. These tumors normally exhibit an elevated internal pressure (turgor) as opposed to their surroundings. This means that a molecule can only reach the tumor interior through diffusion rather than convection. The rate of diffusion directly depends on the size of the molecule, that is, a small recombinant Fv fragment reaches its effector site considerably better than a many times larger IgG.

Alternatively, bispecific Fv antibodies are so small that they are filtered out by the kidneys. Both factors are desirable for the tumor detection in immunoscintigraphy. On the one hand, the tumor is more visible because of the radioactively marked Fv antibody that can enter deep into the tumor. On the other hand, the patient is not unnecessarily burdened with radiation because the radioactively marked Fv antibody is quickly excreted through the kidneys (George et al., 1995).

Attention should be drawn here to another, important difference. In contrast to a bispecific IgG, the corresponding Fv fragments are missing the constant domains (Fig. 1.1). This can also be an advantage in many applications because binding to the Fc receptors, expressed in large quantities on several cells of the immune system, is also suspended. All these properties function together and improve the desired pharmacokinetic properties. As many antibodies as possible should reach their effector site in the tumor interior. As few antibodies as possible should damage healthy tissue due to their nonspecific binding. Unbound antibodies should be excreted as soon as possible (Yokota et al., 1992).

3.3 New Functions Through Heterologous Fusion Partners: Bifunctional Antibodies

3.3.1 WHAT ARE BIFUNCTIONAL ANTIBODIES?

The bispecific antibodies introduced in the previous chapter unite two different antibody specificities in one molecule. Another spectrum of uses is offered by the fusion of an antibody with a heterologous fusion partner, perhaps an enzyme or peptide, a receptor ligand like folic acid, cytokines or a radioactive nuclide. The fusion of whole cells to an antibody by adding a transmembrane domain is also possible. The term "bifunctional antibodies" is used here for artificial molecules with new properties (see Fig. 3.1). They are usually made to attack a tumor directly. As already mentioned, a tumor-specific antibody should concentrate the bifunctional molecule at the tumor, while the heterologous fusion partner supplies the effector functions. When this is a toxin, an immunotoxin results that concentrates at the tumor, and the damage to healthy tissue, to which the antibody cannot bind, is limited (Pastan et al., 1995). Still more refined, is fusion to an enzyme whose activity destroys the tumor. Apart from this, there are many other applications for bifunctional antibodies.

Bifunctional antibodies were also constructed for routine applications in the laboratory, for example, the fusion of Fab' fragments with alkaline phosphatase (Weiss and Orfanoudakis, 1994) or streptavidin (Dübel et al., 1995). Both of these applications offer the added advantage that the affinity to the antigen is increased through dimerization or tetramerization. Antibodies with biotin binding domains can also be used therapeutically. In this way, the selective transport of pharmaceuticals through the blood–brain barrier is made possible by streptavidin conjugates on antitransferrin receptor antibodies (Partridge et al., 1995). Antiganglioside–scFv streptavidin fusions were constructed for radiotherapy (Guo et al., 1996).

3.3.2 BIFUNCTIONAL ANTIBODIES CAN BE USED AS IMMUNOTOXINS

Already briefly discussed in Section 3.2.1.1, a toxin can be transported into the interior of tumor cells by using *bispecific* antibodies. The more direct route is the use of a *bifunctional* antibody, where the toxin is fused directly to a tumor-specific antibody. Compared to the common therapies used today, these immunotoxins represent considerable progress because they selectively detect the cancer cells with the help of their antibody portion and then kill them through the toxic effects. This should produce distinctly fewer side-effects than from the most currently used chemotherapy or radiation therapy, which attack dividing cells relatively nonspecifically. To date, the toxins most frequently fused to antibodies are diphtheria toxin, *Pseudomonas* exotoxin, ricin, saporin, and RNases (reviewed in Reiter and Pastan, 1996; Gottstein et al., 1994).

3.3.2.1 Catalytic Activity: The Key to Potent Toxicity

Many natural toxins inhibit protein synthesis. Diphtheria toxin, for example, transfers an ADP-ribose from NAD^+ to elongation factor eEF2. The eEF2 is thus inactivated. A single molecule of diphtheria toxin can inactivate enough eEF2 molecules to destroy the cell (Lewin, 1996).

Cholera toxin functions differently, it attaches to a central signaling protein of the cell. Similar to diphtheria toxin, the catalytic subunit of cholera toxin transfers ADP-ribose from NAD^+ to the target protein. In this instance, it is the α subunit of the Gs protein, whose function is destroyed by the ADP ribosylation. The Gs protein loses the ability to hydrolyze bound GTP. Thus, the α subunit of the Gs protein is locked in an active state. This in turn activates adenylate cyclase, the result of which is a strongly elevated cAMP level in the cell. The *second messenger* cAMP then regulates the ion channels that are responsible for the symptoms of cholera. It causes the strong outflow of sodium ions and water that lead to the diarrhea typical of cholera (Alberts et al., 1994).

A common feature of these potent toxins is their catalytic activity, that is, only a few of these molecules need to reach the interior of a cell to achieve the devastating effects.

An important prerequisite for the toxic effects of the toxins however, is that their catalytic portion reaches the cytoplasm. This is achieved by most toxins through their modular makeup. One domain of the toxin binds to the receptor on the outside of the cell (for cholera toxin it is the ganglioside GM_1), while another part assists in traversing the plasma membrane, and the third part of the toxin contains the catalytic activity (Choe et al., 1992; Sixma et al., 1992; Li et al., 1996; Zhang et al., 1995).

3.3.2.2 The Binding Domain of a Toxin Can Be Replaced by an Antibody

The key to the design of an immunotoxin lies in the modular structure of the toxins. First, the normal entry of the toxins into the cell interior must, of course, be avoided. This can be achieved by the deletion or mutation of the part of the toxin responsible for the unwanted cell binding. In the next step, the binding domain of the toxin to another target cell is replaced through an antibody fragment and this recombinant toxin is tested for its toxic ability. The aim should be to achieve a destruction by the toxin of only those cells to which the antibody fragment can bind (reviewed in Brinkmann, 1996; see also Brinkmann et al., 1991). Therefore, an antibody fragment that recognizes the tumor cell as specifically as possible is necessary (see also Section 2.3.6.3).

3.3.2.3 Tumor Cells Are Specifically Attacked by Immunotoxins

The immunotoxins have meanwhile proved their effectiveness in many cell culture systems and animal models (reviewed in Pastan et al., 1996; King et al., 1996; see also Kreitman and Pastan 1995; Reiter et al., 1996). A description of the diversity of attempts that have been tried would exceed the scope of this book. Therefore, only a few typical examples can be mentioned here. The *antibody engineering* of the antigen binding site, described in Chapter 2, has been intensively performed especially with immunotoxins, as has the stabilization of Fv fragments with the help of disulfide bridges (Reiter et al., 1994), or the insertion of mutations that improve the affinity, production and the folding of the recombinant antibodies in *E. coli* (Benhar and Pastan, 1995).

The first clinical trials meanwhile report encouraging results on the administering of immunotoxins. In one study, 38 patients with solid epithelial tumors and unsuccessfully treated with conventional therapy, were treated with an immunotxin based on *Pseudomonas* exotoxin. The tumor-specific antibody was directed against the Lewis(y) antigen, a carbohydrate epitope that is overexpressed by many human carcinomas. In five of the 38 patients, a partial remission was observed and one patient even showed a full remission (Pai et al., 1996). The next generation of this immunotoxin will certainly be clinically tested soon. Here, the monoclonal antibody was replaced with a disulfide bridge-stabilized Fv fragment (Kuan et al., 1996).

Only a few of the many other immunotoxins are mentioned here as examples. The fusion of an IgE antibody with the plant toxin ricin led to the long-term ablation of the production of IgE antibodies in a mouse model. Such a bifunctional antibody could be of help to combat serious allergic diseases

(Lustgarten et al., 1996). The ribosome-inactivating protein gelonin was fused to a recombinant anti-CD5 fragment to fight T-cell leukemia cells (Better et al., 1995). Park and colleagues (1995) have followed a somewhat different principle. They coupled a liposome filled with toxin (doxorubicin) to a tumor-specific antibody and thereby achieved a specific destruction of tumor cells.

3.3.2.4 Human Effector Domains: Generation Of Toxicity By Transport Into Another Compartment

All the aforementioned toxins are not of human origin, that is, they can be recognized as foreign by the human immune system. As a result, neutralizing antibodies are formed that erase the desired therapeutic effects after some time (see also Section 2.4.2). For diphtheria toxin, for example, a large number of patients have to be excluded from therapy right from the start because they have already formed a large quantity of neutralizing antibodies due to a diphtheria immunization. The immunotoxins described up to this point therefore allow an administration for only a limited time. Toxins with human origin, which should be barely immunogenic, would be desirable. The use of RNases as a toxic element comes relatively close to this ideal. Many RNases, for example, angiogenin, are found in human serum. When these RNases are coupled to antibodies directed against internalizing antigens, such as the transferrin receptor or the T-lymphocyte antigen CD5, the fusion protein, comprising antibody and RNase, enters the cell and is delivered into the cytoplasm (Fig. 3.6). The RNases unveil their toxic activity that is harmless in the serum (Newton et al., 1992; Zewe et al., 1997). In model systems, this is quite comparable with the above mentioned toxins. As long as the antibody portion

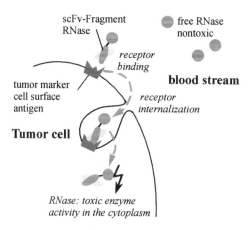

Fig. 3.6.   An immunotoxin combines the cytotoxic effects of a toxin with the selective binding of an antibody. The antibody portion is responsible for the target recognition. Compared to the systemic treatment with cytostatics, the stress on healthy tissue can be considerably reduced. The internalization occurs either through the antibody portion binding of an internalizing surface antigen (e.g., the transferrin receptor) or through special translocation domains from bacterial toxins. The RNase illustrated as an example is nontoxic in its natural compartment. Inside the cell, however, even small amounts are fatal.

of these immunotoxins is of human origin, the goal of a fully human immunotoxin is achieved (Rybak et al., 1992).

The RNases are different from the above mentioned toxins on a second important point. They do not possess their own transport domain that delivers them into the cell interior. As such, the functioning of RNase immunotoxins is still dependent on the recognition of an internalizing antigen. Here a third fusion partner can provide assistance. A transport domain is fused between the RNase and the antibody fragment, for example, an RNase was joined with the domains of *Pseudomonas* exotoxin that are responsible for the recognition and transport (Prior et al., 1992).

3.3.2.5 Nontoxic Substances Can Be Transformed Into Cytotoxins at the Tumor Site

Although immunotoxins could mean a great step forward in the treatment of lymphomas (Gottstein et al., 1994), they still have disadvantages. The main problem is that *all* tumor cells must be killed for a tumor therapy to be successful, otherwise only a little time has been won before the tumor grows anew. Many established tumors are heterogeneous, that is, several tumor cells have lost their tumor-specific antigen and are therefore no longer recognized by the immunotoxin. Theoretically, this can be circumvented by administering several tumor-specific immunotoxins with different antibodies, but another problem remains. Larger molecules have difficulty entering solid tumors. Usually, such tumors have an elevated internal pressure, that is, no molecules can attain the center of a solid tumor by convection, only diffusion is left. This again depends on the size of the molecule. Compared with an IgG, a recombinant immunotoxin can be kept smaller, but even so, it will probably not reach all the cells of a solid tumor. Even smaller molecules would therefore be preferred. Additionally, much would be gained if the tumor-specific toxic element could be successfully broadened to include adjacent cells (*bystander effect*). In this way, the tumor cells that have not bound tumor-specific antibody would also be killed.

This can be achieved with the help of a two component system. First, the tumor-specific antibody searches for its target as described. This time, however, it does not carry the toxic element but an enzyme, which does not otherwise exist in the serum. After some time, the antibody and with it, the enzyme, is concentrated at the site of the tumor. Unbound antibody-enzymes can be excreted from the body. The patient now receives a *prodrug*, a small relatively nontoxic molecule. Through the function of the enzyme, this prodrug is transformed into a toxic substance. Thus, the toxin is only formed where the bifunctional antibody has anchored its enzyme portion, at best, in and around the tumor. Here, it is not important if every tumor cell has been reached by a bifunctional antibody, when the local concentration of the toxin is high enough to destroy all the cells in this area (Fig. 3.7). This technique is called ADEPT (*antibody directed enzyme prodrug therapy*) (reviewed in Bagshaw, 1991; Senter et al., 1993).

All the prodrugs developed to date are very small molecules that can diffuse very quickly into solid tumors. As such, the patient must not be confronted with

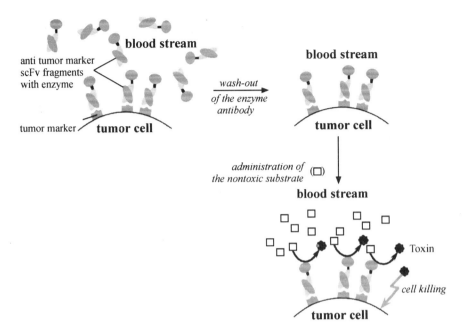

Fig. 3.7. ADEPT: The antibody against the tumor marker does not directly carry a toxic element but an enzyme that is able to generate a toxin at the site of antibody binding after being supplied with a nontoxic precursor (prodrug). The elimination of circulating antibodies before the administration of the prodrug minimizes the side-effects on nonspecific tissue.

potentially toxic substances for long periods, after which they may not even have reached the tumor interior. The partition of the tumor therapy into one phase that is nontoxic for the patient (in which the nontoxic bifunctional antibody reaches the tumor) and a toxic phase (in which the prodrug is transformed into the toxic drug by the enzyme) can be refined still further. Here, all the remaining bifunctional antibodies in the blood stream are inactivated or removed. This is achieved, for example, with a galactose-conjugated antibody against the enzyme portion of the bifunctional antibody. Circulating conjugate is very quickly removed from the blood stream by the liver. The antibody-enzymes that have diffused into the tumor for a long period remain because they are not accessible for the galactose-conjugated antienzyme antibody and are therefore not removed by this step. This reduces the toxic effects on the rest of body even more strongly (Sharma et al., 1994).

One dilemma however remains. The enzymatic portion of the bifunctional antibody should not have a human equivalent. Otherwise, a large background of activated prodrug is to be expected. On the other hand, the enzyme portion should be as human as possible to prevent the formation of inactivating antibodies. Although clinical research is still in its infancy, today several options provide solutions to this problem. One research group has developed a catalytic antibody that transformed a prodrug into an extremely toxic mustard gas (Wentworth et al., 1996). In another model system, the bacterial antibiotic chloramphenicol resulted from the activity of a catalytic antibody

(Miyashita et al., 1993). A further potential solution would be the design of slightly modified human enzymes that have an altered specificity. Human enzymes could also be used that are normally tightly locked inside the cell, in an opposite approach as with RNase, a serum protein whose toxicity is first unveiled in the wrong compartment, the cytoplasm. This requires an enzyme that normally exists only in the cell interior to be combined with a prodrug that cannot traverse the cell membrane. This design has the additional advantage of a positive feedback, that is, a tissue disruption would increase itself due to liberated enzymes from destroyed cells. An example of a successfully used human enzyme is glucuronidase (Bosslet et al., 1994).

3.3.2.6 Antibody–Enzyme Fusions Can Attack Tumors

One of the first, two-component systems used a carboxypeptidase that was chemically coupled to a tumor-specific antibody. This fusion protein did actually concentrate at a previously implanted tumor in an animal model. The addition of the prodrug para-N-bis-(2-choroethyl)aminobenzoylglutamate then led to a selective degradation of the tumor. The prodrug is transformed into a very toxic mustard gas derivative by the carboxypeptidase (Bagshawe et al., 1988).

Another successfully used enzyme for such a process is the bacterial β-lactamase that splits the β-lactam ring of penicillins and cephalosporins. There is no corresponding human enzyme activity, thus no endogenous enzymatic background is expected. First, a prodrug was developed that is transformed into a drug that is 20-fold more toxic (doxorubicin) after the splitting of the β-lactam ring. The two building blocks of the bifunctional antibody were a β-lactamase from *E. coli* and a disulfide bridge-stabilized, humanized Fv fragment directed against the p185[HER2] protoocogene. This antigen is strongly expressed by roughly 30% of breast cancer tumors. This bifunctional antibody could selectively kill breast cancer cells in cell culture (Rodrigues et al., 1995). A very similar approach has even been successfully tested *in vivo*, in a mouse model (Meyer et al., 1993). The human enzyme glucuronidase has also been successfully used in the ADEPT therapy. Mouse models exist in which the bifunctional antibody was bound specifically to a carcinoma (Houba et al., 1996) or the tumor was even destroyed *in vivo* (Bosslet et al., 1994).

3.3.3 RADIOIMMUNOTOXINS

In principle, the local dose of radioactivity at the tumor can be increased, following the two-component principle just described. This was already discussed in Section 3.2.1.2, for which bispecific antibodies were used. Here too, the toxic element (the radiation) also affects the adjacent cells as well as the cells that are bound. This means that tumor should be more selectively and more completely affected. Very encouraging results have already been shown for tumor detection but a considerably higher dose of radiation must be transported to the tumor for a therapy.

The production of bispecific antibodies as described in Section 3.2.1.2 used for tumor detection is comparatively costly. Experimentally, producing monospecific antibodies conjugated to a radioactive substance is much easier. These are also bifunctional according to the definition given in Section 3.3.1. For particular clinical applications, the scFv fragments offer the advantages of a shorter residence time in normal tissue, a quicker removal from the bloodstream and a better penetration of the tumor tissue (Colcher et al., 1990; Milenic et al., 1991; Yokota et al., 1992; Adams et al., 1993; Huston et al., 1993; George et al.,1995; Webber et al., 1995). The following reviews cover this topic: Wawrzynczak and Derbyshire (1992), Goldenberg and Schlom (1993), Goldenberg et al., (1995) and Wilder et al., (1996).

3.3.4 INTRACELLULAR ANTIBODIES

The expression of catalytic antibodies in the cytoplasm of cells was already mentioned in Section 2.4.12. Other recombinant antibodies usually show only a low activity in the cytoplasm. This is probably because antibodies need stabilizing disulfide bridges, which cannot form at a normal rate in the reducing environment of the cytoplasm. In the successful attempts, the antibodies expressed in the cytoplasm usually blocked antigens existing in low amounts. Examples include the enzyme HIV reverse transcriptase (Maciejewski et al., 1995), the G protein *ras* (Werge et al., 1994), and the HIV regulatory protein *rev* (Duan et al., 1994, Wu et al., 1996).

Distinctly more successful was the expression of recombinant antibodies in a more suitable cell compartment: the endoplasmic reticulum (ER). An oxidizing environment dominates here, in which the disulfide bridges important for antibody function can form. Additionally, chaperones are present that are specialized for the correct folding of the immunoglobulins (see also Section 2.1.1). The signal that retains proteins in the ER has been known for several years. It is a small, C-terminal peptide with the core sequence ...KDEL. The same peptide can also confine a recombinant Fab or scFv fragment to the ER. An antibody tagged with ...KDEL can equally restrain an ER-residing antigen in this compartment (Fig. 3.8). The antigen can no longer reach its destination. A "*phenotypic knockout mutant*" develops. The cell carries the antigen gene and the gene product but the latter cannot exercise its function because it is restrained in the wrong compartment by the antibody (Fig. 3.8).

This principle was first shown with envelope protein gp160 from HIV-1. This protein is normally secreted into the ER and then split into two pieces, gp41 and gp120, in the Golgi apparatus. When an scFv fragment specific for the gp160 is simultaneously expressed in the ER, but restrained there through the KDEL sequence, the processing to gp120 and gp41 barely occurs. An anti-*tat* scFv fragment used as a control did not negatively influence the processing. Thus, the production of infectious HIV particles was prevented. Other protein transport through the ER, however, was not disrupted by the scFv fragment (Marasco et al., 1993; Chen et al., 1994). With this method, the blood stem cells essential for survival might one day be rescued from HIV destruction with the help of somatic gene therapy.

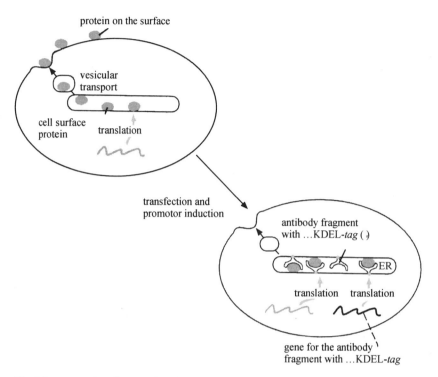

Fig. 3.8.   Production of *somatic knockout mutants* by the expression of antibody fragments with a retention signal for the endoplasmic reticulum (ER).

Tumor cells can also be fought following the same principle. In the given example, a scFv fragment was used against the receptor erbB2. As a result, ovarian carcinoma cells lost the growth signal mediated by this receptor. They stopped their uncontrolled growth and underwent a programmed cell death (apoptosis) (Deshane et al., 1994, 1995a, 1995b). Phenotypic knockouts were also produced for the IL2 receptor in the same way (Richardson et al., 1995).

Plants can also be equipped with a specific "immune system" through the intracellular expression of antibodies, which can protect against viral infection (Tavladoraki et al., 1993), or inactivate a plant hormone such as abscisic acid (Artsaenko et al., 1995).

All these examples illustrate the considerable advantage of the construction of phenotypic knockout mutants in contrast to the previous methodologies: The antibody retained in the ER results in a dominant mutations. Irrespective of where the antibody gene is integrated in the genome, the antibody protein switches off the target antigen. The alternative of completely switching off both alleles of a gene is comparatively more costly (reviewed in Richardson and Marasco, 1995). These advantages are not only limited to cell culture. In the near future, there will probably be a phenotypic knockout mouse that transgenically expresses a scFv fragment. A particularly interesting aspect is that the antibody fragment can be placed under the control of tissue-specific, inducible promoters. This would only retain and and thus inhibit the function of the target antigen in the ER of particular tissues. The use of externally inducible promoters is also possible. The advantage over genetic knockout mutants is especially pertinent, when gene products are important for ontogenesis and when genomic knockouts are lethal, because since the target can be "switched off" at a chosen time point of development.

3.3.5 RECOMBINANT ANTIBODIES CAN BE ANCHORED ON THE SURFACE OF CELLS

Recombinant antibodies can also be directed to other cellular compartments (reviewed in Biocca and Cataneo, 1995). The outer cell membrane is of particular interest. The cell gains an additional property when a recombinant antibody is anchored here. It can bind with other cells or molecules. This can be exploited for cancer therapy, if a cytotoxic T-cell is chosen as the fusion partner of a tumor-specific antibody, with which the antibody binds specifically to the cancer cells and causes them to lyse (Fig. 3.9). This has already worked with two different fusions. T-cells could be activated by the fusion of a scFv

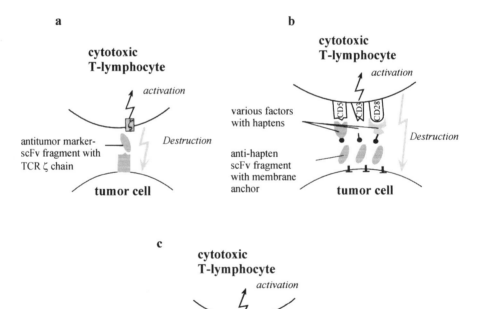

Fig. 3.9. Examples of the expression of antibody fragments on the surface of eukaryotic cells. **(a)** Fusion of a tumor-specific antibody fragment with the ζ chain of the T-cell receptor enables an activation of cytotoxic T-lymphocytes against the tumor cell. **(b)** "Universal" coupling anchor (e.g., against a hapten) (Rode et al., 1996) enables the use of a mixture of signals. **(c)** The expression of an anti-CD28 antibody fragment on a tumor cell allows recognition and destruction by cytotoxic T-lymphocytes.

fragment with the ζ chain of the CD3 complex (Fig. 3.9a). The γ chain of the Fc receptor also seemed suitable as a fusion partner because it is expressed on various immune cells such as *natural killer cells*. Both examples are membrane proteins, which are known to transfer an activation signal to the cytotoxic cells because of their crosslinking. The fusion proteins could seemingly activate the cytotoxic cells after they were crosslinked through the binding of the antigen to a target cell (Eshhar et al., 1993). The T-cells however, require a another signal additional to the crosslinking of the ζ chain because only preactivated T-cells were able to kill the target cells due to the antigen binding. This was shown with the help of a transgenic mouse that expressed the fusion of a Fv fragment with the ζ chain (Brocker and Karjalainen, 1995). Ovarian carcinoma cells (Hwu et al., 1993) and renal carcinoma cells (Weijtens et al., 1996) were similarly lysed by cytotoxic T-cells or mast cells in model systems. Meanwhile, a mouse model exists in which a human ovarian carcinoma was successfully treated (Hwu et al., 1995). Other cells, such as IgE-producing B-lymphocytes, can also be specifically lysed in this way. This could, one day, aid the therapy of serious allergies (Lustgarten and Esher, 1995).

The antibody fragment that mediates the specificity is fused to an effector cell in all these examples. These can actively migrate into tumor tissue so that it is no longer necessary to depend on the passive diffusion of an immunotoxin into the tumor body. One day, this could prove to be a significant and decided advantage in tumor therapy. This is why many laboratories are currently trying to transfect autologous (i.e., of patient origin) effector cells with the DNA that codes for the fusion protein from a tumor-specific scFv fragment and the ζ chain of the CD3 complex. It is still questionable, however, how the once (perhaps overly) - activated effector cells can be switched off again after the successful attack on the tumor.

Concerning this last point, a two-component system, analogous to the universal bispecific antibodies introduced in Section 3.2.4, could help. The cytotoxic effector cells described above would first be transfected with the DNA for a hapten-specific antibody and given back to the patient. Simultaneously, the cancer patient would be injected with tumor-specific antibody that had been previously coupled to the hapten. Only now do these cells attack the tumor, however, only as long as there is supply of the hapten-derivatized, tumor-specific antibody. In this way, the tumor therapy could be steered externally.

Based on a similar idea is the anchoring of a phenyloxazolone (phOx)-specific scFv fragment in the cell membrane (Fig. 3.9b). In this instance, the binding of antigen is not linked with the activational signal on the cell carrying the antibody. The hapten phOx can be very easily coupled to other molecules, as with biotin. Therefore, almost any molecule can be anchored to the surface of cells that express this scFv fragment (Rode et al., 1996). The advantage is that the same cell line can be decorated with many different molecules and even molecule mixtures of various concentrations. For the first time, the influence of several costimulatory molecules on cell lysis, for example, could be systematically quantified, for which cells are decorated with individual or mixtures of antibodies against CD3, CD5, and CD28. In the given example, the relative and absolute quantities of the various antibodies can be varied with ease (Fig. 3.9b).

Moreover, there are still many other conceivable questions. Perhaps an antibody mixture will be found that protects decorated cells from being rejected by the immune system. Enzymes on the surface of tumor cells could perhaps alter their tendency to migrate *in vivo* or the ability to penetrate solid tumors.

It is, of course, also possible to anchor an antibody fragment on the cell surface that directly mediates the costimulatory signal (Fig. 3.9c), for example by binding to the CD28 antigen (Winberg et al., 1996).

3.4 Summary

Antibodies bind with high specifity to their antigens and are therefore essential tools for research and diagnostics. The hybridoma antibodies used until now, however, have not provided comparative success in therapy. Several problems arise in antibody therapy. The production of human antibodies is costly, and binding of a monospecific antibody often does not suffice to activate the immune system. Bispecific antibodies can be obtained by the fusion of two hybridomas. Such bispecific antibodies were already successfully used in several animal models. A Hodgkin lymphoma could be completely healed in a mouse model. Therefore, this method raised hope to obtain highly specific therapeutic reagents against tumors. Recombination of antibodies in microorganisms now allows the construction of a vast variety of fusion proteins with architectures suited to fulfill different tasks. The fusion of two, Fv fragments yields small, *bispecific* antibody fragments that, for many applications, have great advantages over bispecific antibodies obtained from the fusion of two hybridomas. They improve tumor penetration because of their low molecular weight. At the same time, unbound antibodies can be filtered through the kidneys. Both factors together improve the specific signal for tumor detection and thus, also therapy when compared with a native IgG. Other bispecific and bifunctional antibodies bind to tumor cells and mediate a destruction of these cells by activating the immune system. The affinity for an antigen is considerably increased when a bispecific antibody recognizes two adjacent epitopes, compared to the monospecific parental antibodies. Focusing the therapeutic effect to the tumor is therefore possible.

There are very many possibilities for producing bispecific antibodies. A small Fv fragment can be joined to another Fv fragment with the help of a dimerization domain or a cysteine. Fusion with streptavidin leads to tetrameric bispecific antibodies with high affinity for the antigen. Differently placed intermolecular disulfide bridges (in the dsFv fragments) can be exploited for the construction of bispecific antibodies. Diabodies are formed when the variable domains of two scFv fragments are interchanged.

A normal IgG antibody is a molecule with two functions— bifunctional. One function is the specific recognition of the antigen and the other is the activation of the immune system with the help of the constant domains. Gene technology now allows fusion with heterologous binding partners of nearly any origin.

Thus, recombinant bifunctional antibodies allow an enormously extended range of applications, e.g. with the aim of directly attacking a tumor. Here, the tumor-specific antibody portion always has the task of concentrating its fusion partner at the tumor site. The fusion partner can be a radioactive molecule. This enables tumor diagnosis by immunoscintigraphy. Fusion with a toxin yields an immunotoxin. An enzyme concentrated at the tumor can transform a nontoxic precursor substance into one that is toxic and therefore also kill neighboring cells. Several bispecific and bifunctional antibodies have meanwhile reached the stage of clinical trials.

The expression of recombinant antibodies inside a cell can be used to protect the cell from virus infection. It can also cause tumor cells to undergo apoptosis.

References

Adams GP, McCartney JE, Tai MS, Oppermann H, Huston JS, Stafford WF, Bookman MA, Fand I, Houston LL, Weiner LM (1993) Highly specific *in vitro* tumor targeting by monovalent and divalent forms of 741F8 anti-c-*erb*-B-2 single chain Fv. *Cancer Res* **53**:4026–4034.

Alberts B, Bray D, Lewis J, Raff M, Roberts K, Watson JD (1994) Molecular Biology of the Cell, Vol. 3. Garland Publishing, New York, p. 438.

Artsaenko O, Peisker M, zur Nieden U, Fiedler U, Weiler EW, Muntz K, Conrad U (1995) Expression of a single-chain Fv antibody against abscisic acid creates a wilty phenotype in transgenic tobacco. *Plant-J* **8**:745–750.

Bagshawe KD, (1991) Antibody directed enzyme prodrug therapy (ADEPT). Fortner JG, Rhoads JE, editors. Acccomplishments in Cancer Research, Chapman and Hall Medical, London, pp 154–170.

Bagshawe KD, Springer CJ, Searle F, Antoniw P, Sharma SK, Melton RG, Sherwood RF (1988) A cytotoxic agent can be generated selectively at cancer sites. *Br J Cancer* **58**:700–703.

Bakacs T, Lee J, Moreno MB, Zacharchuk CM, Cole MS, Tso JY, Paik CH, Ward JM, Segal DM (1995) A bispecific antibody prolongs survival in mice bearing lung metastases of syngeneic mammary adenocarcinoma. *Int Immunol* **7**:947–955.

Bandtlow C, Schiweck W, Tai HH, Schwab ME, Skerra A (1996) The *Escherichia coli* derived Fab fragment of the IgM/kappa antibody IN-1 recognizes and neutralizes myelin-associated inhibitors of neurite growth. *Eur J Biochem* **241**:468–475.

Benhar I, Pastan I, (1995) Identification of residues that stabilize the single-chain Fv of monoclonal antibodies B3. *J Biol Chem* **270**:23373–23380.

Better M, Bernhard SL, Williams RE, Leigh SD, Bauer RJ, Kung AH, Carroll SF, Fishwild DM (1995) T-cell-targeted immunofusion proteins from *Escherichia coli*. *J Biol Chem* **270**:14951–14957.

Biocca S, Cataneo A (1995) Intracellular immunization: antibody targeting to subcellular compartments. *Trends cell Biol* **5**:248–252.

Bodey B, Siegel SE, Kaiser HE (1996) Human cancer detection and immunotherapy with conjugated and non-conjugated monoclonal antibodies. *Anticancer Res* **16**:661–674.

Bohlen H, Manzke O, Patel B, Moldenhauer G, Dorken B, von Fliedner V, Diehl V, Tesch H (1993a) Cytolysis of leukemic B cells by T-cells activated via two bispecific antibodies. *Cancer Res* **53**:4310–4314.

Bohlen H, Hopff T, Manzke O, Engert A, Kube D, Wickramanayaka PD, Diehl V, Tesch H (1933b) Lysis of malignant B cells from patients with B chronic lymphocytic leukemia by autologous T-cells activated with CD3 × CD19 bispecific antibodies in combination with bivalent CD28 antibodies. *Blood* **82**:1803–1812.

Bosslet K, Czech J, Hoffmann D (1994) Tumor-selective prodrug activation by fusion protein-mediated catalysis. *Cancer Res* **54**:2151–2159.

Brinkmann U (1996) Recombinant immunotoxins: protein engineering for cancer therapy. *Mol Med Today* **2**:439–446.

Brinkmann U, Pai LH, FitzGerald DJ, Willingham M, Pastan I (1991) B3(Fv)-PE38KDEL, a single-chain immunotoxin that causes complete regression of a human carcinoma in mice. *Proc Natl Acad Sci USA* **88**:8616–8620.

Brocker T, Karjalainen K (1995) Signals through T-cell receptor-zeta chain alone are insufficient to prime resting T-lymphocytes. *J Exp Med* **181**:1653–1659.

Carter P, Ridgway J, Zhu Z (1995) Toward the production of bispecific antibody fragments for clinical applications. *J Hematother* **4**:463–470.

Chen SY, Khouri Y, Bagley J, Marasco WA (1994) Combined intra- and extracellular immunization against human immunodeficiency virus type 1 infection with a human anti-gp120 antibody. *Proc Natl Acad Sci USA* **91**:5932–5936.

Choe S, Bennett MJ, Fujii G, Curmi PM, Kantadjieff KA, Collier RJ, Eisenberg D (1992) The crystal structure of diphtheria toxin. *Nature* **357**:216–222.

Colcher D, Bird R, Roselli M, Hardman KD, Johnson S, Pope S, Dodd SW, Pnatoliano MW, Milenic DE, Schlom J (1990) *In vivo* tumor targeting of a recombinant single-chain antigen-binding protein. *J Natl Cancer Inst* **82**:1191–1197.

Cuan L, Bagasra O, Laughlin MA, Oakes JW, Pomerantz RJ (1994) Potent inhibition of human immunodeficiency virus type 1 replication by an intracellular anti-Rev single-chain antibody. *Proc Natl Acad Sci USA* **91**:5075–5079.

Cumber AJ, Ward ES, Winter G, Parnell GD, Wawrzynczak EJ (1992) Comparative stabilities *in vitro* and *in vivo* of a recombinant mouse antibody FvCys fragment and a bisFvCys conjugate. *J Immunol* **149**:120-126.

de Kruif J, Logtenberg T (1996) Leucine zipper dimerized bivalent and bispecific scFv antibodies from a semi synthetic antibody phage display library. *J Biol Chem* **271**:7630–7634.

Demanet C, Brissinck J, De-Jonge J, Thielemans K (1996) Bispecific antibody-mediated immunotherapy of the BCL1 lymphoma: increased efficacy with multiple injections and CD28-induced costimulation. Blood **87**:4390–4398.

Deshane J, Loechel F, Conry RM, Siegal GP, King CR, Curiel DT (1994) Intracellular single-chain antibody directed against erbB2 down-regulates cell surface erbB2 and exhibits a selective anti-proliferative effect in erbB2 overexpressing cancer cell lines. *Gene Ther* **1**:332–337.

Deshane J, Siegal GP, Alvarez RD, Wang MH, Feng M, Caberra G, Liu T, Kay M, Curiel DT (1995a) Targeted tumor killing via an intracellular antibody against erbB-2. *J Clin Invest* **96**:2980–2989.

Deshane J, Caberra G, Grim JE, Siegal GP, Pike J, Alvarez RD, Curiel DT (1995b) Targeted eradication of ovarian cancer mediated by intracellular expression of anti erbB-2 single-chain antibody. *Gynecol Onco* **59**:8–14.

Dübel S, Breitling F, Kontermann R, Schmidt T, Skerra A, Little M (1995) Bifunctional and multimeric complexes of streptavidin fused to single-chain antibodies (scFv). *J Immuno Methods* **178**:201–209.

Dübel, S. (1999) Reconstitution of human RNaseA from two separate fragments fused to different single chain antibody fragments: On the way to binary immunotoxins. Tumor Targeting 4, *in press*.

Ely P, Wallace PK, Givan AL, Graziano RF, Guyre PM, Fanger MW (1996) Bispecific armed, interferon gamma primed macrophage mediated phagocytosis of malignant non Hodgkin's lymphoma. *Blood* **87**:3813–3821.

Eshhar Z, Waks T, Gross G, Schindler DG (1993) Specific activation and targeting of cytotoxic lymphocytes through chimeric single-chains consisting of antibody-binding domains and the gamma or zeta subunits of the immunoglobulin and T-cell receptors. *Proc Natl Acad Sci USA* **90**:720–724.

Fanger MW (1995) Bispecific Antibodies. Springer-Verlag, Heidelberg.

Fanger MW, Graziano RF, Guyre PM (1994) Production and use of anti-FcR bispecific antibodies. *Immunomethods* **4**:72–81.

George AJ, Titus JA, Jost CR, Kurucz L, Perez P, Andrew SM, Nicholls PJ, Huston JS, Segal DM (1994) Redirection of T-cell mediated cytotoxicity by a recombinant single-chain Fv molecule. *J Immunol* **152**:1802–1811.

George AJ, Jamar F, Tai MS, Heelan BT, Adams GP, McCartney JE, Houston LL, Weiner LM, Oppermann H, Peters AM (1995) Radiometal labelling of recombinant proteins by a genetically engineered minimal chelation site: technium 99m coordination by single-chain Fv antibody fusion proteins through a C terminal cysteinyl peptide. *Proc Natl Acad Sci USA* **92**:8358-8362.

Goldenberg D, Schlom J (1993) The coming of age of cancer radioimmunoconjugates. *Immunol Today* **14**:5-7.

Goldenberg DM, Larson SM, Reisfeld RA, Schlom J (1995) Targeting cancer with radiolabeled antibodies. *Immunol Today* **16**:261–264.

Gottstein C, Winkler U, Bohlen H, Diehl V, Engert A (1994) Immunotoxins: is there a clinical value? *Ann Oncol* **5**(Suppl 1):97–103.

Guo HF, Rivlin K, Dübel S, Cheung NKV (1996) Recombinant antiganglioside GD2 scFv-streptavidin fusion protein for tumour targeting. Abstr. of the 1996 annual meeting of AACR (American Association of Cancer Research).

Hakalahti L, Vihko P, Henttu P, Auto-Harmainen H, Soini Y, Vihko R (1993) Evaluation of PAP and PSA gene expression in prostatic hyperplasin and prostatic carcinoma using northern-blot analysis, *in situ* hybridisation and immunohistochimical staining with monoclonal and bispecific antibodies. *Int J Cancer* **55**:590–597.

Hartmann P, Renner C, Jung W, Sahin U, Pfreundschuh M (1996) Treatment of Hodgkin's disease with bispecific antibodies. *Ann Oncol* **7**(Suppl 4):143–146.

Holliger P, Winter G (1993) Engineering bispecific antibodies. *Curr Opin Biotechnol* **4**:446–449.

Holliger P, Prospero T, Winter G (1993) "Diabodies": small bivalent and bispecific antibody fragments. *Proc Natl Acad Sci USA* **90**:6444–6448.

Holliger P, Brissinck J, Williams RL, Thielemans K, Winter G (1996) Specific killing of lymphoma cells by cytotoxic T-cells mediated by a bispecific diabody. *Protein Eng* **9**:299–305.

Houba PH, Boven E, Haisma HJ (1996) Improved characteristics of a human beta-glucuronidase-antibody conjugate after deglycosylation for use in antibody-directed enzyme prodrug therapy. *Bioconjug Chem* **7**:606–611.

Huston JS, McCartney J, Tai MS, Mottola Hartshorn C, Jin D, Waren F, Keck P, Oppermann H (1993) Medical applications of single-chain antibodies. *Int Rev Immunol* **10**:195–217.

Hwu P, Shafer GE, Treisman J, Schindler DG, Gross G, Cowherd R, Rosenberg SA, Eshhar Z (1993) Lysis of ovarian cancer cells by human lymphocytes redirected with a chimeric gene composed of an antibody variable region and the Fc receptor gamma chain. *J Exp Med* **178**:361–366.

Hwu P, Yang JC, Cowherd R, Treisman J, Shafer GE, Eshhar Z, Rosenberg SA (1995) *In vivo* antitumor activity of T-cells redirected with chimeric antibody/T-cell receptor genes. *Cancer Res* **55**:3369–3373.

Janeway CA, Travers P (1997) Immunologie. Spektrum Akademischer Verlag, Heidelberg.

Keyler DE, Sholver WL, Landon J, Sidki A, Pentel PR (1994) Toxicity of high doses of polyclonal drug-specific antibody Fab-fragments. *Int J Immunopharmacol* **16**:1027–1034.

King CR, Fischer PH, Rando RF, Pastan I (1996) The performance of e23(Fv)PEs, recombinant toxins targeting the erbB-2 protein. *Semin Cancer Biol* **7**:79–86.

Kipriyanov SM, Dübel S, Breitling F, Kontermann RE, Little M (1994) Recombinant single-chain Fv-Fragments carrying C terminal cysteine residues: production of bivalent and biotinylated miniantibodies. *Mol Immunol* **31**:1047–1058.

Köhler G, Milstein C (1975) Continuous culture of fused cells secreting antibody of predefined specificity. *Nature* **256**:495–497.

Kostelny SA, Cole MS, Tso JY (1992) Formation of a bispecific antibody by the use of leucine zippers. *J Immunol* **148**:1547–1553.

Kranz DM, Gruber M, Wilson ER (1995) Engineering linear F(ab')2 fragments for efficient production in *Escherichia coli* and enhanced antiproliferative activity. *Protein Eng* **8**:1057–1062.

Kreitman RJ, Pastan I (1995) Targeting *Pseudomonas* exotoxin to hematologic malignancies. *Semin Cancer Biol* **6**:297–306.

Kuan CT, Pastan I (1996) Improved antitumor activity of a recombinant anti-Lewis(y) immunotoxin not requiring proteolytic activation. *Proc Natl Acad Sci USA* **93**:974–978.

Kurucz I, Titus JA, Jost CR, Jacobus CM, Segal DM (1995) Retargeting of CTL by an efficiently refolded bispecific single-chain Fv dimer produced in bacteria. *J Immunol* **154**:4576–4582.

Lamers CH, Gratama JW, Warnaar SO, Stoter G, Bolhuis RL (1995) Inhibition of bispecific monoclonal antibody (bsAb) targeted cytolysis by human antimouse antibodies in ovarian carcinoma patients treated with bsAb targeted activated T-lymphocytes. *Int J Cancer* **60**:450–457.

Lewin B (1998) Gene. Spektrum Akademischer Verlag, Heidelberg.

Li M, Dyda F, Benhar I, Pastan I, Davies DR (1996) Crystal structure of the catalytic domain of Pseudomonas exotoxin A complexed with a nicotinamide adenine dinucleotide analog: implications for the activation process and for ADP ribosylation. *Proc Natl Acad Sci USA* **93**:6902–6906.

Link BK, Weiner GJ (1993) Production and characterization of a bispecific IgG capable of inducing T-cell mediated lysis of malignant B cells. *Blood* **81**:3343–3349.

Little M, Schirrmacher V, Khazaie K, Moldenhauer G, Dübel S, Kypriyanov S, Haas C, Rohde HJ, Gotter S, Breitling F (1994) Bindungsreagenz für Zell Oberflächenprotein und Effektorzelle. Dtsch Pat Reg. Nr. P 1050/133 zi.

Lollo C, Halpern S, Bartholomew R, David G, Hagan P (1994) Noncovalent antibody mediated drug delivery. *Nucl Med Commun* **15**:483–491.

Lustgarten J, Eshhar Z (1995) Specific elimination of IgE production using T-cell lines expressing chimeric T-cell receptor genes. *Eur J Immunol* **25**:2985–2991.

Lustgarten J, Waks T, Eshhar Z (1996) Prolonged inhibition of IgE production in mice following treatment with an IgE-specific immunotoxin. *Mol Immunol* **33**:245–251.

Maciejewski JP, Weichold FF, Young NS, Cara A, Zella D, Reitz MS Jr, Gallo RC (1995) Intracellular expression of antibody fragments directed against HIV reverse transcriptase prevents HIV infection *in vitro*. *Nature Med* **1**:667–673.

Marasco WA, Haseltine WA, Chen SY (1993) Design, intracellular expression, and activity of a human anti-human immunodeficiency virus type 1 gp120 single-chain antibody. *Proc Natl Acad Sci USA* **90**:7889–3793.

McGuinness BT, Walter G, Fitzgerald K, Schuler P, Mahoney W, Duncan AR, Hoogenboom HR (1996) Phage diabody repertoires for selection of large numbers of bispecific antibody fragments. *Nat Biotechnol* **14**:1149–1153.

Meyer DL, Jungheim LN, Law KL, Mikolajozyk SD, Sheperd TA, Mackensen DG, Briggs SL, Starling JJ (1993) Site-specific prodrug activation by antibody-β-Lactamase conjugates: regression and long-term growth inhibition of human colon carcinoma xenograft models. *Cancer Res* **53**:3956–3963.

Milenic DE, Yokota T, Filpula DR, Finkelman MAJ, Dodd SW, Wood JF, Whitlow ML, Snoy P, Schlom J (1991) Construction, binding properties, metabolism and tumor targeting of a single-chain Fv derived from the pancarcinoma monoclonal antibody CC49. *Cancer Res* **51**:6363–6371.

Milstein C, Cuello AC (1983) Hybrid hybridomas and their use in immunohistochemistry. *Nature* **305**:537–540.

Miyashita H, Karaki Y, Kikuchi M, Fujii I (1993) Prodrug activation via catalytic antibodies. *Proc Natl Acad Sci USA* **90**:5337–5340.

Moosmayer D, Dübel S, Brocke B, Watzka H, Hampp C, Scheurich P, Little M, Pfizenmaier KA (1995) Single chain TNF receptor antagonist is an effective inhibitor of TNF mediated cytotoxicity. *Ther Immunol* **2**:31–40.

Müller KP, Kyewski BA (1995) Intrathymic T-cell receptor (TcR) targeting in mice lacking CD4 or major histocompatibility complex (MHC) class II: rescue of CD4 T-cell lineage without co engagement of TcR/CD4 by MHC class II. *Eur J Immunol* **25**:896–902.

Neri D, Momo M, Prospro T, Winter G (1995a) High affinity antigen binding by chelating recombinant antibodies (CRAbs). *J Mol Biol* **246**:367–373.

Neri D, de Lalla C, Petrul H, Neri P, Winter G (1995b) Calmodulin as a versatile Tag for Antibody Fragments. *Biol Technol* **13**:373–377.

Newton DL, Hercil O, Laske DL, Oldfield E, Rybak SA, Youle RJ (1992) Cytotoxic ribonuclease chimeras. *J Biol Chem* **267**:19572–19578.

Nisonoff A, Rivers MM (1961) Recombination of a mixture of univalent antibody fragments of different specificity. *Arch Biochem Biophys* **93**:460–462.

Orfanoudakis G, Karim B, Bourel D, Weiss E (1993) Bacterially expressed Fabs of monoclonal antibodies neutralizing tumour necrosis factor alpha *in vitro* retain full binding and biological activity. *Mol Immunol* **30**:1519–1528.

Pack P, Kujaru M, Schroeckh V, Knupfer U, Wenderoth R, Riesenberg D, Plückthum A (1993) Improved bivalent miniantibodies, with identical avidity as whole antibodies, produced by high cell density fermentation of *Escherichia coli*. *Biotechnol NY* **11**:1271–1277.

Pai LH, Wittes R, Setser A, Willingham MC, Pastan I (1996) Treatment of advanced solid tumors with immunotoxin LMB-1; an antibody linked to Pseudomonas exotoxin. *Natl Med* **2**:350–353.

Pardridge WM, Boado RJ, Kang YS (1995) Vector-mediated delivery of a polyamide ("peptide") nucleic acid analogue through the blood-brain barrier *in vivo*. *Proc Natl Acad Sci USA* **92**:5592–5596.

Park JW, Hong K, Carter P, Asgari H, Guo LY, Keller GA, Wirth C, Shalaby R, Kotts C, Wood WI (1995) Development of anti-p185HER2 immunoliposomes for cancer therapy. *Proc Natl Acad Sci USA* **92**:1327–1331.

Pastan IH, Pai LH, Brinkmann U, Fitzgerald DJ (1995) Recombinant toxins: new therapeutic agents for cancer. *Ann NY Acad Sci* **758**:345–354.

Pastan I, Pai LH, Brinkmann U, Fitzgerald D (1996) Recombination immunotoxins. *Breast Cancer Res Treat* **38**:3–9.

Peltier P, Curtet C, Chatal JF, Le Doussal JM, Daniel G, Aillet G, Gruaz-Guyon A, Barbet J, Delaage M (1993) Radioimmunodetection of medullary thyroid cancer using a bispecific anti-CEA/anti-indium-DPTA antibody and an indium-111-labeled DPTA dimer. *J Nucl Med* **34**:1267–1273.

Perisic O, Webb PA, Hollinger P, Winter G, Williams RL (1994) Crystal structure of a diabody, a bivalent antibody fragment. *Structure* **2**:1217–1226.

Prior TI, FitzGerald DJ, Pastan I (1992) Translocation mediated by domain II, of *Pseudomonas* exotoxin A: transport of basnase into the cytosol. *Biochemistry* **31**:3555–3559.

Raag R, Whitlow M (1995) Single-chain Fvs. *FASEB J* **9**:73–80.

Reiter Y, Pastan I (1996) Antibody engineering of recombinant Fv immunotoxins for improved targeting of cancer: disulfide stabilised Fv immunotoxins. *Clin Cancer Res* **2**:245–252.

Reiter Y, Brinkmann U, Jung SH, Lee B, Kasprzyk PG, King CR, Pastan I (1994) Improved binding and antitumor activity of a recombinant anti-erb B2 immunotoxin by disulfide stabilization of the Fv-Fragment. *J Biol Chem* **269**:18327–18331.

Reiter Y, Wright AF, Tonge DW, Pastan I (1996) Recombinant single-chain and disulfide-stabilized Fv-immunotoxins that cause complete regression of a human colon cancer xenograft in nude mice. *Int J Cancer* **67**:113–123.

Rheinneckar M, Hardt C, Ilag LL, Kufer P, Gruber R, Hoess a, Lupas A, Rottenberger C, Plückthum A, Pack P (1996) Multivalent antibody fragments with high functional affinity for a tumor associated carbohydrate antigen. *J Immunol* **157**:2989–2997.

Richardson JH, Marasco WA (1995) Intracellular antibodies: development and therapeutic potential. *Trends Biotechnol* **13**:306–310.

Richardson JH, Sodroski JG, Waldmann TA, Marasco WA (1995) Phenotypic knockout of the high-affinity human interieukin 2 receptor by intracellular single-chain antibodies against the alpha subunit of the receptor. *Proc Natl Acad Sci USA* **92**:3137–3141.

Rode HJ, Little M, Fuchs P, Dörrsam H, Schooltink H, de Ines C, Dübel S, Breitling F (1996) Cell surface display of a single-chain antibody for attaching polypeptides. *Biotechniques* **21**:650, 652–653, 655–658.

Rodrigues ML, Presta LG, Kotts CE, Wirth C, Mordenti J, Osaka G, Wong WL, Nuijens A, Blackburn B, Carter P (1995) Development of a humanized disulfide-stabilized anti-p185HER2 Fv-beta-lactamase fusion protein for activation of a cephalosporin doxorubicin prodrug. *Cancer Res* **55**:63–70.

Rybak SM, Hoogenboom HR, Meade HM, Raus JC, Schwartz D, Youle RJ (1992) Humanization of immunotoxins. *Proc Natl Acad Sci USA* **89**:3165–3169.

Sahin U, Tureci O, Schmitt H, Cochlovius B, Johannes T, Schmits R, Stenner F, Luo G, Schobert I, Pfreundschuh M (1995) Human neoplasma elicit multiple specific immune responses in the autologous host. *Proc Natl Acad Sci USA* **92**:11810–11813.

Schumacher J, Klivenyi G, Matys R, Stadler M, Regiert T, Hauser H, Doll J, Maier-Borst W, Zoller M (1995) Multistep tumor targeting in nude mice using bispecific antibodies and a gallium chelate suitable for immunoscintigraphie with positron emission tomography. *Cancer Res* **55**:115–123.

Segal DM, Sconocchia G, Titus JA, Jost CR, Kurucz I (1995) Alternative triggering molecules and single-chain bispecific antibodies. *J Hematother* **4**:377–382.

Senter PD, Wallace PM, Svensson HP, Vrudhula VM, Kerr DE, Hellström I, Hellström KE (1993) Generation of cytotoxic agents by targeted enzymes. *Bioconjugate Chem* **4**:3–9.

Sharma SK, Bagshawe KD, Burke PJ, Boden JA, Rogers GT, Springer CJ, Melton RG, Sherwood RF (1994) Galactosylated antibodies and antibody-enzyme conjugates in antibody-directed enzyme prodrug therapy. *Cancer* **73**(3 Suppl):1114–1120.

Shelver WL, Keyler DE, Lin G, Mustaugh MP, Flickinger MC, Ross CA, Pentel PR (1996) Effects of recombinant drug-specific single chain antibody Fv fragment on [3H]-desipramine distribution in rats. *Biochem Pharmacol* **51**:531–537.

Sixma TK, Pronk SE, Kalk KH, van Zanten BAM, Berghuis AM, Hol WGJ (1992) Lactose binding to heat-labile enteroxin revealed by X-ray crystallography. *Nature* **355**:561–564.

Somasundaram C, Matzku S, Schumacher J, Zöller M (1993) Development of a bispecific monoclonal antibody against a gallium-67 chelate and the human melanoma-associated antigen p97 for potential use in pretargeted immunoscintigraphy. *Cancer Immunol Immunother* **36**:337–365.

Tavladoraki P, Benvenuto E, Trinca S, De Martinis D, Cattaneo A, Galeffi P (1993) Transgenic plants expressing a functional single-chain Fv antibody are specifically protected from virus attack. *Nature* **366**:469–472.

Tazzari PL, Zhang S, Chen Q, Sforzini S, Bolognesi A, Stirpe F, Xie H, Moretta A, Ferrini S (1993) Targeting of saporin to CD25-positive normal and neoplastic lymphocytes by an antisaporin/anti-CD25 bispecific monoclonal antibody: *in vitro* evaluation. *Br J Cancer* **67**:1248–1253.

Wawrzynczak EJ, Derbyshire EJ (1992) Immunotoxins: the power and the glory. *Immunol Today* **13**:381–383.

Webber KO, Kreitman RJ, Pastan I (1995) Rapid and specific uptake of anti-Tac disulfide-stabilized Fv by interleukin-2 receptor-bearing tumors. *Cancer Res* **55**:318–239.

Weijtens ME, Willemsen RA, Valerio D, Stam K, Bolhouis RL (1996) Single-chain Ig/gamma gene-redirected human T-lymphocytes produce cytokines, specifically lyse tumor cells, and recycle lytic capacity. *J Immunol* **157**:836–843.

Weiner LM, Clark JI, Ring DB, Alpnugh RK (1995a) Clinical development of 2B1, a bispecific murine monoclonal antibody targeting c erbB2 and Fc gamma RIII. *J Hematother* **4**:453–456.

Weiner LM, Clark JI, Davey M, Li WS, Garcia de Palazzo I, Ring DB, Alpaugh RK (1995b) Phase I trial of 2B1, a bispecific monoclonal antibody targeting c erbB2 and Fc gamma RIII. *Cancer Res* **55**:4586–4593.

Weiss E, Orfanoudakis G (1994) Application of a alkaline phosphatase fusion protein system suitable for efficient screening and production of Fab-enzyme conjugates in *Escherichia coli. J*

Biotechnol **33**:43–53.

Weiss E, Chatellier J, Orfanoudakis G (1994) *In vivo* biotinylated recombinant antibodies: construction, characterization, and application of a bifunctional Fab-BCCP fusion protein produced in *Escherichia coli. Protein Expr Purif* **5**:509–517.

Wentworth P, Datta A, Blakey D, Boyle T, Partridge LJ, Blackburn GM (1996) Toward antibody-directed "abzyme" prodrug therapy, ADAPT: carbamate prodrug activation by a catalytic antibody and its *in vitro* application to human tumor cell killing. *Proc Natl Acad Sci USA* **93**:799–803.

Werge TM, Baldari CT, Telford JL (1994) Intracellular single-chain Fv antibody inhibits Ras activity in T-cell antigen receptor stimulated Jurkat cells. *FEBS Lett* **351**:393–396.

Wickham TJ, Segal DM, Roelvnik PW, Carrion ME, Lizonova A, Lee GM, Kovesdi I (1996) Targeted adenovirus gene transfer to endothelial and smooth muscle cells by using bispecific antibodies. *J Virol* **70**:6831–6838.

Wilder RB, DeNardo GL, DeNardo SJ (1996) Radioimmunotherapy: recent results and future directions. *J Clin Oncol* **14**:1383–1400.

Winberg G, Grosmaire LS, Klussman K, Hayden MS, Fell HP, Ledbetter JA, Mittler RS (1996) Surface expression of CD28 single-chain Fv for costimulation by tumor cells. *Immunol Rev* **153**:6–14.

Wu Y, Duan L, Zhu M, Hu B, Kubota S, Bagasra O, Pomerantz RJ (1996) Binding of intracellular anti-Rev single-chain variable fragments to different epitopes of human immunodeficiency virus type 1 rev: variations in viral inhibition. *J Virol* **70**:3290–3297.

Yokota T, Milenic DE, Whitlow DE, Whitlow M, Schlom J (1992) Rapid tumor penetration of a single-chain Fv and comparison with other immunoglobulin forms. *Cancer Res* **52**:3402–3408.

Zewe M, Rybak SM, Dübel S, Coy JF, Welschof M, Newton DL, Little M (1997) Cloning and cytotoxicity of a human pancreatic RNase immunofusion. *Immunotechnology* **3**:127–136.

Zhang RG, Scott DL, Westbrook ML, Nance S, Spangler BD, Shipley GG, Westbrook EM (1995) The three-dimensional crystal structure of cholera toxin. *J Mol Biol* **251**:563–573.

Zhu Z, Lewis GD, Carter P (1995) Engineering high affinity humanized anti-p185HER2/anti CD3 bispecific F(ab')2 for efficient lysis of p185HER2 overexpressing tumor cells. *Int J Cancer* **62**:319–324.

Chapter 4
Production and Purification of Recombinant Antibody Fragments

4.1 Properties of Recombinant Antibodies and Choice of Expression System

The breakthrough for the technology of recombinant antibodies was mainly aided by the emergence of the new selection systems in *E. coli* (see also Section 2.3.5). It became clear very quickly, however, that *E. coli* was not always the most suitable organism for *production*. Despite the high homology between various antibodies, the efficiency of production and folding could vary by several orders of magnitude (Orfanoudakis et al., 1993). This finding is not surprising, however, because even in homologous expression systems (myeloma cell lines), single point mutations in the hypervariable regions can dramatically influence the formation and secretion of antibodies (Chen et al., 1994).

The quantities yielded from *E. coli* are usually sufficient for an initial analysis of the specificity and affinity. Additionally, the great strength of selection methods conducted in *E. coli* lies in their high throughput. To obtain a larger quantity of antibodies however, the production usually has to be optimized first by changing to other expression systems or by targeted modifications of the folding properties of the antibody fragment. However, since the effort of changing the expression system is usually justified only after performing an initial characterization of the recombinant antibody fragment, thus *E. coli* expression systems still have their place.

In the two following sections, several expression systems for recombinant antibody fragments will be introduced. First, a few definitions must be explained.

4.1.1 STRUCTURAL CHARACTERIZATION OF AN ANTIBODY: THE DEFINITION OF THE HYPERVARIABLE REGIONS (CDRs)

A standardized numbering system for the individual amino acid residues is required to enable a comparison of the primary structures of various antibodies. Through such comparisons, for example, the germline genes from which the antibody originated can be found, or sequence modifications brought about by somatic hypermutation can be identified.

The heterogeneity in the length of the hypervariable regions causes definition problems. The length of the CDR3 of the heavy chain can vary from 4 to more than 20 amino acid residues, for example. Additionally, various structural definitions of the synonymously used terms "hypervariable region" and "CDR" exist. Already evident from the term, the original categorization of the hypervariable regions is exclusively based on the comparison of various antibody sequences. This is represented in the Kabat databank of immunological molecules (Kabat et al., 1987). A system for numbering the amino acid residues in the variable regions was introduced based on the existing sequence data at that time. This Kabat numbering scheme enables an easy comparison of various antibodies and is therefore widely used. With the growing number of known sequences, however, additional amino acid positions had to be inserted. The reason for this being the length polymorphism of the hypervariable regions just mentioned. The inserted positions received letters in addition to the position number. The amino acid positions of the variable domains from Kabat are presented in Table 4.1. The positions of the hypervariable areas are emphasized in bold.

Table 4.1   The Numbering of the Amino Acid Residues of the Variable Regions

Light chain

0	1	2	3	4	5	6	7	8	9
10	11	12	13	14	15	16	17	18	19
20	21	22	23	**24**	**25**	**26**	27		
27A	**27B**	**27C**	**27D**	**27E**	**27F**			28	29
30	**31**	**32**	**33**	**34**	35	36	37	38	39
40	41	42	43	44	45	46	47	48	49
50	**51**	**52**	**53**	**54**	**55**	**56**	57	58	59
60	61	62	63	64	65	66	67	68	69
70	71	72	73	74	75	76	77	78	79
80	81	82	83	84	85	86	87	88	89
90	**91**	**92**	**93**	**94**	**95**				
95A	**95B**	**95C**	**95D**	**95E**	**95F**	**96**	**97**	98	99
100	101	102	103	104	105	106			
106A	107	108	109						

Heavy chain

0	1	2	3	4	5	6	7	8	9
10	11	12	13	14	15	16	17	18	19
20	21	22	23	24	25	26	27	28	29
30	**31**	**32**	**33**	**34**	**35**				
35A	35B					36	37	38	39
40	41	42	43	44	45	46	47	48	49
50	**51**	**52**							
52A	**52B**	**52C**	**53**	**54**	**55**	**56**	**57**	**58**	**59**
60	**61**	**62**	**63**	**64**	**65**	66	67	68	69
70	**71**	**72**	73	74	75	76	77	78	79
80	81	82							
82A	82B	82C	83	84	85	86	87	88	89
90	91	92	93	94	**95**	**96**	**97**	**98**	**99**
100									
100A	**100B**	**100C**	**100D**	**100E**	**100F**	**100G**	**100H**	**100I**	**100J**
100K	**101**	**102**	103	104	105	106	107	108	109
110	111	112	113						

The Kabat numbering system was used (Kabat et al., 1987).
Some antibodies have insertions exceeding the numbers as given above. No standard nomenclature is used in these cases. Table according to Andrew Martin.

In contrast, the term *complementarity-determining regions* (CDR) is defined from the binding to the antigen. A whole range of crystal structure data has become available since the characterization of the hypervariable regions. They show that the actual binding sites are not exactly in agreement with the hypervariable regions. It was also soon clear that the inserted positions of the Kabat definition did not correspond to the structurally correct insertion points. Therefore, a modified numbering system was introduced that corrected for this, called the Chothia numbering method (Chothia and Lesk, 1987). The numbering of the amino acid residues in the Chothia system was, in principle, exactly the same as that in the Kabat system, except that the additional amino acid residues were inserted at a different place. The amino acid positions of the variable domains according to Chothia are presented in Table 4.2. The positions of the CDRs are emphasized in bold.

Table 4.2   The Numbering of the Amino Acid Residues of the Variable Regions

Light chain

0	1	2	3	4	5	6	7	8	9
10	11	12	13	14	15	16	17	18	19
20	21	22	23	**24**	**25**	**26**	**27**	**28**	**29**
30									
30A	**30B**	**30C**	**30D**	**30E**	**30F**				
	31	**32**	**33**	**34**	35	36	37	38	39
40	41	42	43	44	45	46	47	48	49
50	**51**	**52**	**53**	**54**	**55**	**56**	57	58	59
60	61	62	63	64	65	66	67	68	69
70	71	72	73	74	75	76	77	78	79
80	81	82	83	84	85	86	87	88	89
90	**91**	**92**	**93**	**94**	**95**				
95A	**95B**	**95C**	**95D**	**95E**	**95F**	**96**	**97**	98	99
100	101	102	103	104	105	106			
106A	107							108	109

Heavy chain

0	1	2	3	4	5	6	7	8	9
10	11	12	13	14	15	16	17	18	19
20	21	22	23	24	25	**26**	**27**	**28**	**29**
30	**31**								
31A	**31B**								
		32	33	34	35	36	37	38	39
40	41	42	43	44	45	46	47	48	49
50	51	52							
52A	**52B**	**52C**	**53**	**54**	**55**	**56**	57	58	59
60	61	62	63	64	65	66	67	68	69
70	71	72	73	74	75	76	77	78	79
80	81	82							
82A	82B	82C	83	84	85	86	87	88	89
90	91	92	93	94	**95**	**96**	**97**	**98**	**99**
100									
100A	**100B**	**100C**	**100D**	**100E**	**100F**	**100G**	**100H**	**100I**	**100J**
100K	**101**	**102**	103	104	105	106	107	108	109
110	111	112	113						

The Chothia numbering system was used (Chothia and Lesk, 1987). Table according to Andrew Martin.

Table 4.3   Comparison of the Numbering Methods for the V Regions (according to A. Martin)

CDR	Kabat	Numbering Scheme Chothia	Contact	
L1	L24 › L34	L24 › L34	L30 › L36	
L2	L50 › L56	L50 › L56	L46 › L55	
L3	L89 › L97	L89 › L97	L89 › L96	
H1	H31 › H35B	H26 › H32...34	H30 › H35B	(Kabat method) or
H1	H31 › H35	H26 › H32	H30 › H35	(Chothia method)
H2	H50 › H65	H52 › H56	H47 › H58	
H3	H95 › H102	H95 › H102	H93 › H101	

H, heavy chain; L, light chain.
Compilation by Andrew Martin. Taken from his excellent web site at:
http://www.biochem.ulc.ac.uk/ ~martin/abs/GeneralInfo.html#kabatnum
The end of the CDR-H1 according to Chothia varies, depending on the distance between H32 and H34, when it is numbered according to Kabat because in the Kabat method insertions at H35A and H35B are made as follows: when either 35A or 35B exists, the CDR-H1 ends at 32; when only 35A exists, the CDR-H1 ends at 33; when 35A and 35B exist, the CDR-H1 ends at 34.

The definition of the amino acid positions by MacCallum et al., (1996) refers to CDRs more consistently. It is based entirely on the analysis of the actual antigen contacts from structural data. This "contact" numbering method is not yet widely used. Its advantages become especially evident if the candidate amino acids participating in antigen binding are determined through a sequence comparison with other antibodies. This can be very important for the design of a library based on random sequences (see also Sections 2.2.8 and 2.2.9), or in the mutagenesis of an existing antibody to improve its affinity (see also Section 2.4.7 and following). Table 4.3 compares the three numbering systems, in which each of the six regions important for antigen binding is presented.

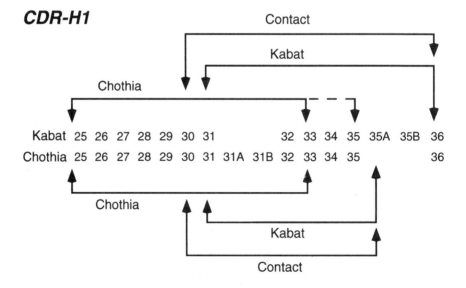

Fig. 4.1. Numbering of the amino acid residues of the CDR1 of the heavy chain according to various authors. According to Andrew Martin. Find more information on his excellent web site at: http://www.biochem.ucl.ac.uk/~martin/abs/GeneralInfo.html#kabatnum

The consequences are presented in more detail in Figure 4.1 using the example of the CDR-H1. Comprehensive data on CDR structure, antibody sequence organization and the CDR-antigen contacts can be obtained from the Internet under http://www.biochem.ucl.ac.uk/~martin/abs/MeanContacts.html

It should not be forgotten however, that the amino acid residues that directly participate in antigen contact are not solely responsible for the shape, and thus, for the specificity or affinity of the antibody. Residues further away can also substantially participate in the determination of the conformation of the CDR loops and so dramatically influence the specificity and affinity (Hawkins et al., 1993, Liu et al., 1999).

4.1.2 BIOCHEMICAL CHARACTERIZATION OF AN ANTIBODY: SPECIFICITY AND AFFINITY

In addition to the antigen-independent factors that determine the shelf-life, such as stability against proteases or against spontaneous denaturing, there are two important antigen-dependent properties that judge the usefulness of an antibody. They are its specificity and its affinity. They are a measure of the quality of an antibody with respect to antigen binding. Both are determined by the structure of the antibody's site of contact with the antigen.

4.1.2.1 What Is Specificity?

The *specificity* indicates how well an antibody can distinguish between different antigen structures. On a molecular level, it is determined by the interactions between the variable chains and the antigen. Two protein surfaces come into contact that should match each other as well as possible. This then determines the amount and strength of the noncovalent, intermolecular bonds formed upon antigen contact. The shape of the surface and the arrangement of these bonds are mainly responsible for the specificity, while the type and energy contribution of these bonds are important factors for the *affinity*.

When another molecule incidentally has a surface similar to the antigen against which the antibody is made, and can additionally form similar intermolecular bonds, a *cross-reaction* of the antibody with this molecule results. Cross-reactions are frequently observed between homologous proteins from different species, whose amino acid sequences are barely distinguishable. However, completely different proteins with no sequence homology can also be recognized by the same antibody. For example, an antibody raised against a neuropeptide (EPPGGSKVILF) also binds strongly to another protein that shows no sequence homology at all to this epitope (Keppel and Schaller, 1991). In another example, two peptides with completely different sequences bound with similar high affinity (dissociation constants in the nanomolar range) to one antibody. Analysis of the crystal structure showed that both peptides existed in completely different structures, and partly interacted with different portions of the antigen binding site (Schneider-Mergener, personal communication).

4.1.2.2 Cross-Reaction and Nonspecific Binding

A cross-reaction of a monoclonal antibody or a recombinant antibody fragment should not be confused with its *nonspecific binding*. The two interactions differ in the type of bond (Fig. 4.2). A cross-reaction is mediated, by definition, through the antigen binding site (the *idiotype*) and often possesses affinities that are similar to the antigen binding. Therefore, in an attempt to suppress the unwanted side reaction, removal of cross-reactive antibodies in an experimental setting by preincubation with the nonspecific antigen is not possible. This is possible, however, with a polyclonal serum in which antibodies can exist that are against other epitopes of the same antigen. Nonspecific binding, in contrast, is mediated by other portions of the molecule. Examples include adhesion to plastic surfaces in ELISA, to the nitrocellulose of an immunoblot or to membrane remnants and to denatured protein aggregates in cell or tissue staining. To avoid this type of binding, the nonspecific binding sites can be blocked by an excess of other proteins. Frequently used are 1–5% (w/v) serum albumin, 3% (w/v) collagen (gelatin), or 0.5–2% (w/v) casein (milk powder).

A further source of nonspecific binding is denatured antibodies. Antibodies denature through frequent freeze/thawing (especially in diluted solutions) or by strong heating. Hydrophobic amino acid residues from the antibody interior reach the surface and then bind nonspecifically to the substrate. An incubation with some nonionic detergents (e.g., Nonidet NP40, Tween 20, Triton X-100) that mask the hydrophobic surfaces with a polar layer can often be of help.

In cell or tissue staining, the Fc receptors on some cell surfaces can also cause nonspecific binding to the constant domains of the antibody. This problem can be avoided by incubating with an excess of other antibodies Fc fragments or the application of Fab' or scFv fragments. Cross-reactions and nonspecific binding in antibodies to be used for *in vivo* therapeutic purposes or in diagnosis present a particular problem. There is no general solution for this. Each individual antibody must be accurately tested for corresponding side effects.

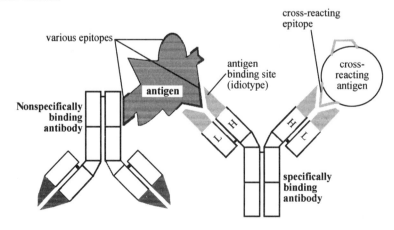

Fig. 4.2.   Some terms to describe antibody–antigen reactions (related to the antigen).

4.1.2.3 The Structure of the Epitope: a Key Feature for the Usefulness of Antibodies

Information about the structure of the antigen epitope is of practical help. The *epitope* is the portion of the antigen that interacts on a molecular level with the antibody. There is a distinction between haptens (small, organic compounds that are often bound by a cavity formed by the hypervariable domains) and larger epitopes. Binding to a protein is usually mediated by a larger epitope. An antibody can bind to a single section of the polypeptide strand (sequential epitope). These antibodies also usually bind with comparable affinity to oligopeptide fragments (5–15 amino acid residues) from the protein sequence, which correspond to the sequential epitope (see below).

When amino acid residues contribute to the binding which are not directly following each other on the polypeptide chain, this is known as a conformational epitope. Amino acid residues from different parts of the protein chain or even from different proteins in a multimer can constitute an epitope. A special subgroup of conformational epitopes are the *local* epitopes which are composed of secondary structures. A typical example is the alphabetical epitope, where every second to third residue contributes to the binding (Liu et al., 1999; Kneissel et al., 1999). Binding to such larger epitopes is possible because the hypervariable domains can form a protein surface up to 750 $Å^2$.

There is no rule, however, about how many of the six hypervariable domains share in the antigen binding. As such, antibodies have been described in which only the heavy chain is required for antigen binding (Ward et al., 1989; Barry and Lee, 1993), or at least substantially determine the specificity (Brigido et al., 1993; Song et al., 1997). In other antibodies, CDR's on both chains have been identified to be essential for binding (Liu et al., 1999).

The type of epitope has practical consequences for the usefulness of an antibody in various immunoassays. Some conformational epitopes are irreversibly destroyed by denaturation of the antigen. Therefore, such epitopes can no longer be recognized by the antibody on a Western blot after denaturing SDS gel electrophoresis. Different fixing methods in cell staining (ethanol treatment, aldehyde fixation) can also destroy protein epitopes. Some antibodies that recognize conformational epitopes do not bind, or only weakly, to an isolated oligopeptide because this corresponds only to a portion of the antigen. Local alpha-helical epitopes, however, can sometimes retain their structure in SDS gel electrophoresis. In conclusion, the epitope structure has to be evaluated for every antibody individually to allow conclusions on its interaction with the antigens.

4.1.2.4 What is Affinity?

The strength of the binding of an antibody to its antigen, its affinity, is the second important factor in evaluating the quality of an antibody. The strength of this binding is given by its binding constant. The binding constant is a measure of the reaction equilibrium that arises between the antigen-bound and the antigen-dissociated antibody molecules. The more antibody that exists in equilibrium in the antigen bound state, the better the affinity of the antibody for its antigen.

4.1.2.5 Determination of the Affinity by Equilibrium Analysis

Ideally, this equilibrium is measured experimentally, where both partners occur in solution. First, an equilibrium or steady state is allowed to form, that is, until as many bonds are formed as are dissolved. Then, the free antibodies are separated from those bound and each quantity is determined. The binding constant (dissociation constant K_d) is calculated according to a formula derived from the law of mass action:

$$\frac{x}{a} = \frac{1}{K_d}(i_{tot} - x)$$

where
$$x = \text{bound antibody}$$
$$a = \text{free antigen}$$
$$i = \text{free antibody}$$
$$i_{tot} = \text{total antibody}$$
$$a_{tot} = \text{total antigen}$$

and
$$a = a_{tot} - x$$
$$x = i_{tot} - i.$$

The separation of free and bound antibody can be achieved by centrifugation or equilibrium filtration (Fazekas de St Groth and Webster, 1961; Hardie and Van Regenmortel, 1975). There are also methods in which one partner is bound to a solid phase, such as the surface of an ELISA plate. The binding constants obtained in this way, however, often deviate considerably from those obtained in solution (Lethonen, 1981; Underwood, 1985). This is because proteins can be partially denatured by binding to the plastic surface and additionally, may adhere in a way that the epitope is no longer accessible. Therefore, the use of methods that allow for the initial binding equilibrium to establish in solution has to be preferred. Thereafter, the amount of unbound antibody can be determined by an ELISA. Here, a separation of the bound from the unbound antibody is not necessary, if establishing a new equilibrium in the detection ELISA is not given too much time. This is achieved through short incubation periods and a limited amount of antigen on the solid phase. Both factors require that a maximum of 10% of the total amount of the *free* antigen binds to the ELISA plate (and thereby removed from the equilibrium). Fulfilment of this condition can be measured by first adding the equilibrium mixture of antigen and antibody to an ELISA plate containing antigen. After a defined time, the samples are taken out again and pipetted into new ELISA wells. They should be incubated for exactly the same time as for the previous assay and the amount of bound antibody is determined for both. The difference between both values should not exceed 10% (Friguet et al., 1985), otherwise the measured values for the equilibrium constant are substantially affected by the assay system. Further possibilities for providing the affinity constant can be used for particular antigens, depending on their properties. Examples include the fluorescence quench method or stop-flow methods, both of which cause a change in the light absorption, fluorescence or other biochemical properties as a result of binding (Bashford and Harris, 1988).

4.1.2.6 Determination of the Affinity Through the Direct Measurement of Association and Dissociation

The binding equilibrium (K_a) can also be described kinetically as a ratio of the association rate (*on-rate*, k_{ass}) and the dissociation rate (*off-rate*, k_{diss}):

$$K_a \quad = \quad \frac{k_{ass}}{k_{diss}}$$

A modern method for determining the binding constant is based on a direct determination of these kinetic constants. This is possible with instruments that through surface plasmon resonance (BIAcore) show the loading of a surface with a number of molecules in real time. When a solution of antibodies flows over such a surface, to which the antigen is coupled, a saturation curve is obtained for the increase in mass. When the antibody solution is removed, the bound antibody molecules begin to detach from the antigen. A second curve is obtained for the loss of mass after the removal of antibody from the solution. The association and dissociation rates can be directly determined from each curve and thereby their ratio, the binding constant.

Newer experiments however, indicate that the effect of the rebinding can yield artificially elevated values for the affinities. Depending on the antibody concentration, a measured deceleration of the dissociation is thus obtained that pretends a higher affinity, according to the equation above. This phenomenon is countered experimentally by the addition of an excess of soluble antigen and/or a minimization in the amount of antigen during the measuring phase of the dissociation rate.

Most recently, binding properties of recombinant antibodies have been assessed while the antibody fragment is still being presented on the surface of a phage (see Section 2.3.4). A mass sensitive microsensor method allows the determination of antibody affinity directly from the phage supernatant, thus making possible a 'high throughput' affinity comparison of a large number of specifically binding clones as they are frequently obtained from a phage panning (see Section 2.3.5). Binding of phage antibodies to antigen immobilised on a Quartz Crystal Microbalance (QCM) induces a mass dependent decrease in frequency. This principle was employed to determine the binding constant of a scFv (single chain) antibody against RNA Polymerase of Drosophila melanogaster presented on the surface of an filamentous phage (M13) from its association and dissociation rates (Hengerer et al., 1999). The obtained affinity is in accordance with the affinity of the scFv fragment as determined by the conventional equilibrium ELISA and plasmon resonance methods. The quantity of phage particles required for a set of measurements can easily be generated in a small scale lab culture, thus saving the time consuming steps of subcloning/transformation in a separate expression system and the preparation and purification of the antibodies from the bacteria.

4.1.2.7 Avidity: The Number of Binding Sites Affects the Binding Constant

On a molecular level, the value of the binding constant is determined by the sum of the atomic interactions between hypervariable domains of the variable chains and the antigen. These interactions are dependent on the pH value, the temperature and the salt concentration of the surrounding medium. Ideally, each of these conditions should be included when stating the binding constant. Usually, the affinities of antibodies are determined at 25°C in physiological saline at pH 7.0–7.6. Additionally, the determination method used must always be considered when stating the binding constant. Fluctuations of the obtained affinity between various measurements are possible as a result. Comparisons of antibody affinities are therefore most reliable when the binding constants were determined in the same experiment.

An important reason for the continual discrepancies in affinity determinations is the different *avidities* of antibodies. A natural IgG molecule possesses two identical antigen-binding sites, and therefore, a higher avidity compared with only one binding site in a recombinant scFv or Fab' fragment. This difference leads to considerable variations in the measured affinity, depending on which of the assays is used. When, due to the setup, many antigen molecules lie close together, that is, in the reach of both arms of the IgG, this molecule can be tightly held with both arms. In another assay, where less antigen is used, the IgG can only bind with one arm. The dissociation of the antibody from the antigen is now easier, and the antibody appears suddenly to have a lower affinity for its antigen.

This avidity effect is exploited by nature. In the first antibody immune response to a new antigen there are no antibodies available that have undergone somatic hypermutation and therefore have an improved affinity. To compensate for this, the body uses IgM molecules. These are composed of five antibody "Ys" joined at their Fc portions. Thus, 10 identical antigen binding sites are united in one molecular complex. In this way, new antigens can be marked with sufficient affinity through hypervariable domains, despite binding that is not yet optimized. The differences in the determined affinity, between the whole molecular complex and the single monovalent antigen binding site, can come to several orders of magnitude for IgM molecules (Roggenbuck et al., 1994; Ciric et al., 1995). A whole range of methods has been developed in recombinant antibody technology to obtain an affinity increase with the help of dimer oligomerization of single scFv or Fab' fragments (see also Sections 3.2.3 and 3.3.1 and the following)

Examples named here are the fusions of scFv fragments to *core* streptavidin (Dübel et al., 1995) or to the tetramerization domain of the human transcription factor p53 (Rheinecker et al., 1996).

4.1.2.8 Different Applications of Antibodies Require Different Affinities

Affinities in the micromolar range are required for practical applications in everyday laboratory immunoassays such as immunofluorescence, ELISA, or immunoblots. Natural antibodies with very high affinities achieve binding constants of 10^{10} $1 \times mol^{-1}$. Sometimes, such a high affinity is undesirable, e.g., when antibodies have to be employed for the affinity chromatographic purification of an antigen. The stronger the binding, the more stringently the column must be eluted, with the risk that the antigen or the antibody is thereby denatured. For such applications, antibodies with affinities of roughly 10^6 $1 \times$ mol^{-1} are better. Despite the relatively low affinity of the antibody for its antigen, the function of affinity chromatography is nearly quantitative because the high concentration of the antibody (compared with the antigen concentration) on the column shifts the equilibrium in favor of binding. It is therefore possible to use this method successfully to enrich an antigen with antibodies which only weakly react on immunoblots or in cell staining.

4.1.3 DIFFERENT APPLICATIONS OF ANTIBODIES REQUIRE DIFFERENT EXPRESSION SYSTEMS

The optimal folding and glycosylation conditions are most likely provided in descendants of immune system cells because these are responsible for the antibody production in the body. For example, if an antibody is to bind the complement component C1q or the cell surface receptor FcγR, a correct glycosylation at ASN 297 of the CH2 region is necessary. When, however, as often happens, only the actual antigen binding is needed, the effort of mammalian cell culture can be spared. Expressing the scFv or Fab fragments in yeast or bacteria might be sufficient.

Production in transgenic animals or plants would only make sense when particularly large amounts of correctly glycosylated antibodies are required, or for use *in situ* in the creation of somatic knockout mutants (Brocker and Karjalainen, 1995; Piccioli et al., 1995) (see also section 3.3.4).

Sometimes, it must simply be tested in which expression system an antibody can be expressed at all. An scFv fragment has been described which could be expressed in *E. coli* and in a Baculovirus system but not in mammalian cell lines (Brocks et al., 1997). In Table 4.4, several expression systems for recombinant antibody fragments are categorized with respect to these laboratory-relevant characteristics. In the following two sections, these systems are discussed in detail.

4.2 Prokaryotic Expression Systems

4.2.1 PRODUCTION IN *E. COLI*

E. coli is the "workhouse" of modern molecular biology. Correspondingly, there is no other organism for which there is nearly as much experience in the

Table 4.4   **Various Systems for the Production of Recombinant Antibody Fragments**

Organism	Growth	Transformation	Yield	Glycosylation[*]
In vitro				
Reticulocyte lysate (rabbit)	Not necessary	Not necessary	Very low	No
Prokaryotic organisms				
E. coli				
Cytoplasm	Very fast	Simple	High/S–S refolding necessary	No
Soluble fraction of the periplasma	Very fast	Simple	Low – medium	No
Periplasmatic inclusion bodies	Very fast	Simple	High/ refolding necessary	No
Gram-positive				
Bacillus	Fast	Simple	High[+]	No
Streptomyces	Fast	Simple	High[+]	No
Eukaryotic organisms				
Yeast (*Pichia, Saccharomyces, Schizosaccharomyces*)	Medium	Arduous	Variable[+]	Partial
Trichoderma	Medium	Arduous	High[+]	Partial
Baculovirus (insect cells)	Medium	Not too arduous	Variable to high	Partial
Mammalian cells (myeloma, CHO, COS)	Medium	Arduous	Variable to high	Yes
Transgenic plants (tobacco)	Very slow	Very arduous	High[+]	Partial
Transgenic animals	Very slow	Very arduous	High[+]	Yes

[*] The type of glycosylation is very important for some biological functions of the antibody. A fully correct glycosylation only occurs in mammalian cells.
[+] In these systems a general estimate is not possible due to the few existing examples.

expression of different proteins. Depending on the choice of expression vector, the possibility exists to obtain soluble recombinant proteins from the cytoplasm, from cytoplasmic or periplasmic inclusion bodies, or from the periplasmic space. The latter is the space between the two membranes that build the outer coat of the bacterium together with the proteocglycan layer it includes. Occasionally, recombinant proteins can also be obtained from the culture medium.

4.2.1.1 The Yield of Recombinant Antibody Fragments Is Not Predictable

The *E. coli* cell is not suitable for producing complete IgG molecules. Fab' fragments that are roughly twice the size of scFv fragments are produced, but often, with low yields (Skerra and Plückthun, 1991). The mutation of a single codon can also dramatically influence the expression in *E. coli* (Duenas et al., 1995; Knappik and Plückthun, 1995; Ulrich et al., 1995). A study with 512 mutants of a Fv fragment showed that more than 10%, random point mutations in the CDRs could hinder the production in *E. coli* (Ito et al., 1993). Many recombinant antibodies can apparently not be folded correctly in *E. coli*. The reverse also applies in that the yield can be dramatically increased by modifications to a few amino acids.

The actual constraint in the production of recombinant antibody fragments in *E. coli*, according to these studies, lies apparently in the folding of the correct tertiary structure. This can currently only be helped by modifications in the antibody sequence itself (Knappik and Plückthun, 1995). Several "key points" could be identified in the framework areas that drastically influenced the folding efficiency. The coexpression of additional folding helpers (Knappick et al., 1993) has not led to any remarkable change in the yield of functional proteins so far.

One or several of these factors could therefore cause the potential appearance of differences in yields of soluble proteins of several orders of magnitude between recombinant antibody fragments with very similar sequences. Empirically, Fab' or scFv fragments that were selected from phage libraries, were produced in *E. coli* with higher yields of soluble protein than those obtained from hybridoma lines. This might be because antibody fragments that are produced well are also more easily incorporated into the surface of the phage particle (see also Sections 2.3.4 and 2.4.9). During the antigen screening, this leads to a preference for those antibody genes that are produced at a higher rate and/or are folded more correctly in the *E. coli* periplasma. A selection with phage libraries therefore always also includes a selection according to production ability in *E. coli* (Deng et al., 1994) (see also Section 2.4.9).

4.2.1.2 Fab' Fragments or scFv Fragments?

Complete antibodies such as an IgG have not been successfully produced in *E. coli* so far because the folding apparatus of *E. coli* is apparently overtaxed. Thus, the choice remains between expression as a Fab' fragment or as a scFv fragment. Fab' fragments are usually more stable than scFv fragments but the yield is lower from *E. coli*. ScFv fragments however aggregate at high concentrations (see Section 2.4.9).

The yield of Fab' fragments can be increased, within limits, by modification of the mRNA secondary structure (Stremmer et al., 1993), but the actual constraint in the production of functional antibody fragments is the compatibility with the secretion and folding mechanisms of the *E. coli* cell. For example, a significant improvement in the secretion of a Fab' fragment could be achieved by the exchange of the light chain (Cκ replaced by Cλ) (MacKenzie et al., 1994). The constant regions of the Fab' fragment offer the advantage that cheap, commercial antisera against light/heavy chains can be used for their detection. Additionally, established methods of purification from classical antibody technology can be used (see Section 4.4.3.3). The constant regions that only exist in Fab' fragments are responsible for the major contribution of binding energy between the two antibody chains, in particular, through a disulfide bridge. This is the reason for the comparatively high stability of the Fab' fragments.

This bond, which stabilizes the variable region is missing in scFv fragments. However, Fv fragments can also be artificially stabilized by the insertion of disulfide bridges at the contact surfaces between the regions (see Section 2.4.10) (Glockshuber et al., 1990; Brinkmann et al., 1993).

The small scFv fragments were predicted to be advantageous in a whole range of *in vivo* applications due to their short residence time in tissue, a quicker removal from the circulation and a better penetration of tumor tissue (Colcher et al., 1990; Milenic et al., 1991; Yokota et al., 1992; Adams et al., 1993; Huston et al., 1993) (see also Section 3.2.1.2). In the neutralization of the antidepressive drug, desipramine, the scFv fragments were removed more quickly from the blood but were more stable in serum than the corresponding Fab' fragments (Shelver et al., 1996).

A systematic comparison of various recombinant antibody fragments, directed against the carcinoembryonic antigen (CEA, a marker used for tumor detection), gave the following results. Monomeric scFv fragments were filtered out from the blood by the kidneys too quickly. As such, a significant dose could not bind to the tumor tissue. Dimerizing the scFv antibodies caused 15% of the material to be found in the tumor tissue. The best effect, however, was given by a construct three times the size of the monomer. It comprised two scFv fragments held together through a CH3 dimer. In contrast, even larger F(ab)$_2$ fragments and complete IgG antibodies bound less well to the tumor tissue by comparison (Wu et al., 1996). Smaller antibody fragments (Fab' and scFv) apparently effect a more even binding to tumor tissue than that of complete IgG (Buchsbaum, 1995). Another study, using chemical conjugates of the tumor marker B72.3, yielded the following results. Mono/di/trimeric coupling of scFv fragments resulted in an unsatisfactory concentration at the tumor. By contrast, dimerized and trimerized Fab' molecules showed a better tumor-specific concentration (King et al., 1994). In conclusion, it is evident that the influence of the construct size on the pharmacokinetic parameters has to be evaluated for each antigen-antibody pair individually.

4.2.1.3 Intracellular Expression Requires *In Vitro* Folding

High expression yields were achieved in the first studies on the expression of recombinant Fab' fragments in *E. coli*. The Fab' fragments formed were denatured and stored in cytoplasmic inclusion bodies. A costly renaturation of the denatured antibody fragments had to be carried out first, so that functional antibodies could be obtained from this system. In the given example, only roughly 1% of the produced fragments could be folded into functional Fab' fragments (Cabilly et al., 1984). This method is not suitable for producing large amounts of Fab' fragments, although advances have been made meanwhile in *in vitro* folding, and the yield could be increased to 60 µg/ml (Buchner and Rudolf, 1991). Better results have been obtained with monomeric scFv fragments than with the heterodimerized proteins Fab' or Fv. In some cases, even the incorrect folding of the proteins was of use because this allowed the production of extremely toxic proteins. Examples include fusions of recombinant antibody fragments to *Pseudomonas* exotoxin (Spence et al., 1993) or to a human RNase (Zewe et al., 1997). This method can also provide advantages for particular antibody sequences as opposed to the secretion systems introduced in the next section. The soluble expression of a scFv fragment against the human complement component C5 did not lead to useful yields, while 8% (12.5 mg/l) of functional antibodies could be obtained through their refolding from the cytoplasm from a total production of 150 mg/l of culture medium (Evans et al., 1995).

In a few cases, the expression of low quantities of soluble functional antibody fragments in the cytoplasm of *E. coli* was described (Proba et al., 1995). Some other special cases are referred to in Sections 2.4.12. The reducing environment of the cytoplasm however, hinders the efficient production of soluble, functional antibody fragments.

4.2.1.4 Secretion Into The Periplasma Allows a Correct Folding of Antibody Fragments

Two studies published in 1988 showed that antibody fragments were secreted through the internal membrane of *E. coli* and could fold into functional molecules in the periplasma (Better et al., 1988; Skerra and Plückthun, 1988). This was achieved by the fusion of a bacterial signal peptide to both antibody chains. In contrast to the cytoplasm, an oxidizing environment dominates in the periplasma of *E. coli* that enabled the correct formation of the disulfide bridges in the antibody chains (Glockshuber et al., 1992).

Comparisons of affinity and the production quantities showed that a large proportion of the soluble recombinant antibodies from the periplasma could be folded into functional proteins (Kazemier et al., 1996). Periplasmatic secretion is currently the most frequently used method for the production of recombinant antibodies for initial laboratory testing. Its particular advantages are that a complete cell lysis is not required because a periplasmatic protein fraction can easily be obtained that is already highly enriched.

4.2.1.5 Genetic Elements of Secretion Vectors for *E. coli*

A range of excellent laboratory manuals exists in which the methods for the expression and purification of recombinant proteins from *E. coli* are described in detail (e.g., Harris and Angal, 1989; Sambrook et al., 1989). Here, only a few examples can be mentioned on the influence of genetic elements on cloning and expression of recombinant antibodies. For the expression of toxic proteins, it is crucial to use a highly repressible promoter that only allows for expression after induction. Otherwise, a selection pressure results that is too strong for the expression of the recombinant protein, and thus, the danger of inactivating mutations arises. In our hands, the expression of a fusion protein from scFv fragments with streptavidin was only possible with the help of a synthetic promoter that could be very tightly regulated (Dübel et al., 1995). The same applied to the stable cloning of an RNase gene (M. Zewe, personal communication). Another suitable vector system used a tetracycline promoter that could be very tightly repressed but chemically induced (Schiweck and Skerra, 1995).

The sequence of the ribosomal binding site also influences the amount of expression. An improved production of a scFv fragment was achieved through a *random* mutagenesis of the ribosomal binding site (Wilson et al., 1994).

A prerequisite for the secretion of the recombinant antibody chains is the fusion to signal peptides recognised by the *E. coli* secretion apparatus, which allows translocation from the cytoplasm into the periplasma. The signal sequences from the genes *pelB, ompA, ompF, EcPhoA,* or *stII* used so far show no great differences in the yield of recombinant antibodies (Somerville et al., 1994). In one report, a roughly 10-fold improvement in the yield was achieved through a mutation in the signal peptide sequence. This effect however, could be traced back to an altered secondary structure of the mRNA (Stemmer et al., 1993). Yields of 0.01–40 mg/l were achieved from shaking cultures using a range of various vectors in a laboratory setting (Better and Gavit, 1997). The use of cultures containing extremely high cell densities (an OD_{550} of up to 100 was achieved that translates into more than 10^{11} cells per milliliter) in fermenters. Here, up to 1 mg/ml and more of recombinant antibody fragments can be obtained with secretion systems (Tai et al., 1990; Carter et al., 1992; Better et al., 1993; Pack et al., 1993). Notice should always be taken, however, of the fact that the yield of a particular recombinant antibody fragment does not imply conclusions about the efficiency of production of another. As mentioned above, the primary sequence and the folding efficiency determine the yield.

Only a small portion of the total functional protein is secreted by fermenting cultures. As such, Carter and coworkers (1992) could obtain 100 mg/l of a Fab' fragment from fermentation culture medium. A yield of 2 g/l was achieved after ultrasound sonification. An improvement in the yield of soluble protein can be achieved through induction by low temperatures in most cases (Gandecha et al., 1992). A variety of studies suggested a range of 24–32°C to be optimal. Often, however, the largest fraction of proteins produced in this way was accumulated in an insoluble form.

The strength of the induction also influences the relationship of correctly folded to insoluble antibody fragments. An induction of the promoter that is too strong overtaxes the secretion apparatus and does not lead to a further increase in the amount secreted (Dübel et al., 1992). Lowered expression was even observed by induction that was too strong (Sawyer et al., 1994).

The duration of promoter induction also affects the yield of recombinant antibody fragments. A short time (2-3 hours) following induction, the expression of some antibodies led to bacterial lysis (Fuchs et al., 1991, Froyen et al., 1993). In this instance, proteases are liberated that can reduce the yield of functional antibodies. The lytic effect of a scFv fragment could be eliminated by fusion to a bacterial proteoglycan-associated lipoprotein. This fusion, however, caused a fraction of the secreted protein to bind to the cell wall (Fuchs et al., 1991).

4.2.1.6 *In Vitro* Folding of Recombinant Antibody Fragments

Despite the advantages of *E. coli* secretion vectors in the routine laboratory, they are seldom suitable for the production of large quantities. This is particularly true for toxic recombinant proteins such as the immunotoxins introduced in Section 3.3.2. Such proteins can be produced in large amounts (up to 30% of the total cell protein) in *E. coli* in the form of inclusion bodies. The yield of function-competent recombinant proteins now depends on the most efficient method possible for refolding these denatured proteins (e.g., Reiter et al., 1996; Ross et al., 1996). Periplasmic inclusion bodies have advantages for refolding of antibody fragments because the disulfide bridges can be formed more easily in this compartment (Kipriyanov et al., 1994).

One advantage of renaturing bacterial inclusion bodies comprises an initial very easy and efficient purification step. Directly following cell lysis, the inclusion bodies are separated from the total soluble proteins by centrifugation. This is followed by repeated washing of the inclusion bodies with moderate concentrations of nonionic detergents. The methods described for refolding then usually use a chaotropic agent to solubilize the inclusion bodies, for example, 8 M urea and/or 6 M guanidinium chloride. Refolding is allowed by a gradual dilution of the denaturing agents, usually by dialysis (Kipriyanov et al., 1994). Alternatively, this can also occur by the gradual addition of the denatured antibody fragments to a renaturation solution (Buchner et al., 1992a). Problems often occur in *in vitro* folding of recombinant antibody fragments when too high a concentration of recombinant antibody fragments is used during the folding process. This leads to the aggregation of proteins that are not yet fully renatured. A concentration step is therefore recommended only after the renaturation, at best, even after an additional purification of the monomer by size exclusion chromatography. The use of weakly destabilizing agents, such as arginine, has proved to be helpful in the renaturation of recombinant antibody fragments in neutral or weakly alkaline pH during the refolding process.

Some publications report that the addition of chaperones like GroEL or protein disulfide isomerase leads to improved folding efficiencies (Buchner et al., 1992b; Duenas et al., 1994). These methods are still the subject of controversy (Lah et al., 1994; Humphreys et al., 1996). A conclusive statement is probably not possible at this time because of the incomplete knowledge about the very complex chaperone system that serves to fold the immunoglobulins correctly in the body.

4.2.1.7 The Orientation of the Variable Regions in scFv Fragments Can Influence Production

The order in which the variable regions follow each other in a scFv polypeptide strand can strongly influence the yield of functional protein. The order of preference in which the domains are produced is not predictable however. In one instance the order VH-linker-VL was better, in another it was reversed (see below). The majority of recombinant antibody fragments so far have been produced in the orientation VH-linker-VL, with only a few in the reversed orientation.

The influence of the orientation of the variable domains on production was only investigated systematically in a few cases. For a scFv fragment against a *Salmonella* surface protein, a very similar amount of polypeptide was produced in both orientations (ca. 50 mg/ml) but only correctly secreted and folded to a small extent. The proportion of the correct product amounted to roughly 5% of the total protein for the construct with the VH-linker-VL orientation, while the opposite orientation yield was 20-fold lower (Anand et al., 1991). The orientation also had a similar influence on a scFv fragment against ovalbumin lysozyme (Tsumoto et al., 1994). The reversed orientation proved to be advantageous for the secretion of a scFv fragment against hepatitis B virus antigen. The reason for this could be narrowed down as follows. An arginine in the framework 1 region of the heavy chain, near to the signal sequence, disrupted the passage of the polypeptide through the membrane. After its exchange for a glycine, the VH-linker-VL construct could also be produced (Ayala et al., 1995). The rule also applies here that the optimal orientation for each scFv fragment must be determined separately.

4.2.2 PRODUCTION IN GRAM-POSITIVE BACTERIA

The gram-positive bacteria *Bacillus subtilis* offers one advantage over *E. coli*. Proteins secreted through the cell membrane can freely diffuse into the surrounding medium because there is no second, outer cell membrane that encloses the proteoglycan sacculus. True secretion is an exception in *E. coli*. Here, the scFv and Fab' fragments are retained by the outer membrane in the periplasma.

Unfortunately, the molecular methods for cloning foreign genes into *Bacillus* are not established to the same extent as for *E. coli*. The secretion of proteases through the *Bacillus* cells has also represented a long-standing problem because many proteins are destroyed as soon as they are successfully secreted into the medium. Laboratory strains now exist with considerably reduced protease activity. As such, up to 5 mg/l culture of scFv fragments have been obtained in shaking flask cultures of *Bacillus subtilis* in a laboratory setting (Wu et al., 1993).

Another gram-positive bacterium, the euactinomycete *Streptomyces lividans*, was also used successfully in the recombinant reproduction of Fv fragments. Using a homologous promoter and the *Streptomyces* subtilisin-inhibitor signal sequence, yields of up to 1mg/l culture could be achieved, of which the majority could bind and inactivate antigen (ovalbumin lysozyme) (Ueda et al., 1993).

Due to the particular culture requirements and the less well known genetics of these organisms, they have not been able to dominate over established systems such as *E. coli*, insect or mammalian cells, despite their theoretical advantages.

4.3 Eukaryotic Expression Systems for Recombinant Antibodies

As already discussed in Section 4.2.1.2, antibody fragments are more poorly produced as their size increases in *E. coli*. The yield of Fab's is usually lower than that for Fv or scFv fragments, and complete IgG molecules are practically not formed at all. Therefore, the only option for the production of complete IgG molecules is eukaryotic cells.

4.3.1 EXPRESSION IN THE CYTOPLASM

Practically all eukaryotic expression systems for recombinant antibody fragments use the secretory pathway. The special case '*intracellular antibodies*,' that is, expression in the cytoplasm or with retention signals for the endoplasmic reticulum or the cell surface, are not used for mass production and were discussed in Sections 3.3.4 and 3.3.5.

4.3.2 THE CELLS OF THE IMMUNE SYSTEM ARE THE NATURAL PRODUCTION SITES FOR ANTIBODIES

In the body, the vast majority of antibodies is produced by plasma cells. These circulate as single, mobile cells in the blood and can secrete large amounts of immunoglobulins. The secretion of antibodies begins with passage of both antibody chains through the membrane of the endoplasmic reticulum. The immunoglobulin chains are provided with a signal sequence for this process that is proteolytically removed after passage through the membrane. In the endoplasmic reticulum, the chains are folded, laid together and the *intra-*, like the *inter-*, chain disulfide bonds are formed. A whole range of different helper factors and chaperones are involved in this process, such as the immunoglobulin heavy-chain-binding protein (BiP or GRP78) or protein disulfide isomerase (PDI) that help in the formation of the disulfide bridge bonds. The constant domains are then glycosylated by passage through the Golgi apparatus before secretory vesicles provide transport to the cell surface. Therefore, plasma cells should be especially suitable for the production of recombinant antibodies. Plasma cells however, cannot be cultivated easily *in vitro*. Plasma cell descendants and their precursors, the B cells, offer an alternative after they are immortalized by transformation into tumor cells. Therefore, expression in plasmacytoma and myeloma cell lines is the closest possible variation to the natural situation for the production of recombinant antibodies. These cells provide the whole set of help mechanisms, such as the right chaperones in the endoplasmic reticulum or the correct glycosylation mechanisms. The cell's own antibody genes must, of course, be inactivated beforehand because heterogenous mixtures, containing only a small proportion of the desired antibody, would otherwise result (see also Section 3.2.1 and Fig. 3.3).

Two different vector concepts were developed for eukaryotic expression. Transient expression is the easier and quicker method. It merely requires the transformation of the cells with episomal DNA, analogous to *E. coli* expression. The disadvantage is that not all the cells are transfected and moreover, the amount produced can vary greatly. Additionally, such expression vectors are usually not stable for longer periods. To achieve the latter, a stable integration of the antibody gene into the genome of the cell line is needed (stable transfection). A large number of commercial vectors are available for both applications. Various recombinant antibodies were expressed in plasmacytoma cells (Conrad et al., 1991) or myeloma cell lines. These cells are suitable for the production of Fab' fragments (Bender et al.,1993), Fv fragments

(King et al.,1993) or scFv fragments (Kitchin et al., 1995) and equally for the new types of constructs. An example is a recombinant antibody fragment in which a scFv fragment was fused to the *hinge*-region of the heavy chain (Shu et al., 1993; Qi and Xiang, 1995). In this case, murine SP2/0 myeloma cells were used. Even the polycistronic expression of chimeric mouse/human IgG molecules succeeded under the control of a bacterial promoter system (T7) in SP2/0 cells (Deyev et al., 1993). The generation of peritoneal tumors (ascites method) is also possible with these cells, which have been used to obtain large amounts of antibodies by monoclonal antibody technology (Werge et al., 1992).

4.3.3 PRODUCTION IN OTHER MAMMALIAN CELLS

4.3.3.1 COS Cells

Vectors for COS cells have the SV40 *origin of replication*. COS cells were originally obtained from the kidneys of monkeys and express the *large T antigen* of the SV40 virus, which is responsible for the efficiency of replication. Therefore, high numbers of copies of the plasmids are achieved inside the COS cells that produce the large SV40 T antigen. For many years, COS cells have been preferentially used for transient expression, that is, for the expression of episomal DNA that is not integrated into the genome. The use of COS cells is then always prudent, when a fast and uncomplicated system is needed for the production of antibody fragments without stable integration, for example for the screening of mutants or to test new types of constructs (e.g., Morton et al., 1993; Ridder et al., 1995a). Murine Fab' fragments obtained from a phage library could be simply produced and characterized in the form of a complete IgG molecule in COS cells (Ames et al., 1995). More complicated constructs such as a bispecific (scFv)$_2$ fusion composed of an OKT3-scFv fragment and an anti-human transferrin receptor scFv were also successfully produced in COS cells (Jost et al., 1996). Here, the amount produced was not lower than that of the singly produced scFv fragments. This shows the advantage over *E. coli*, where the expression of such tandem constructs is often low or even not possible.

COS cells glycosylate the recombinant antibody fragments produced. This glycosylation promotes secretion into the culture medium (Jost et al., 1994). In the same study, the functional proportion of antibodies secreted from COS cells was determined to be more than 90%.

4.3.3.2 *Chinese Hamster Ovary (CHO) Cells*

A derivative of CHO cells contains in its genome an RNA polymerase gene of the bacteriophage T7 equipped with the nuclear localization signal of the large SV40 T antigen. Thus, protein production can be regulated via transcription from the efficient T7 promoter. The achievable yields are in the range of mg/ml in lab scale cultures (King et al., 1993; Dorai et al., 1994). In the case of a bispecific antibody from two scFv fragments, one against the CD3 antigen of human T-cells and the other against the epithelial 17-1A antigen from colorectal cancer cells, expression of a functional product was successful only in CHO cells but not in *E. coli* (Mack et al., 1995).

CHO cells can also be used for the production of stably transfected cell lines. In this instance, the amount produced can be increased by coselection with metabolic markers. The yield was successfully increased from 0.5 mg/ml to 200 mg/ml through several dihydrofolate reductase (dhfr) amplification steps (Page and Sydenham, 1991). Genetic heterogeneity however, was also observed in stable cell lines (Harris et al., 1993). Applicable here, as for conventional monoclonal antibodies, is the need for the frequent control of antibody production and, if necessary, frequent subcloning.

4.3.4 PRODUCTION OF RECOMBINANT ANTIBODY FRAGMENTS IN INSECT CELLS (BACULOVIRUS SYSTEM)

The original baculovirus system comprised *Spodoptera frugiperda* (Sf-9) insect cells and baculoviruses that could be cultivated with ease in the laboratory (reviewed Matthews, 1982). The production and secretion of heterologous proteins is achieved through the infection with recombinant *Autographa californica* nuclear polyhedrosis virus (AcNPV) or related viruses. The system has already been used for the heterologous expression of a variety of different proteins (reviewed in Maeda, 1989). The advantages of this system lie in a high transformation efficiency, a large yield of secreted proteins and simple culture. Additionally, for recombinant antibodies produced for therapeutical use, no risk exists of a contamination with mammalian pathogenic viruses.

Insect cells are comparatively closely related to mammalian cells so that many human proteins can be correctly folded in these cells, probably due to chaperones that can take over the functions of BiP and other native helper proteins. These cells also recognize the signals for *N*-glycosylation although they differ from mammalian cells in the composition of sugar chains (Jarvis et al., 1990).

To obtain recombinant proteins from insect cells, the DNA for the recombinant antibody fragment is first cloned into an *E. coli* transfer vector. These vectors carry an *E. coli origin of replication*, in addition to the baculovirus portion, and code for an antibiotic resistance gene for selection in *E. coli*. Thus, the formation of the antibody gene occurs in such a way that its expression is driven by very strong insect promoters. A frequently used promoter is that of the polyhedrin, a protein that is necessary for the formation of a type of *long-lived spores* (occlusion bodies), but not for the normal infection pathway. After the identification of a correct, recombinant, transfer vector clone, its DNA, together with incomplete viral DNA, is cotransformed into insect cells, usually with the calcium phosphate method. The transfer vector expression cassette recombines with the viral DNA in the insect cells and forms a function-competent baculovirus, so that the formation of virus particles can occur. Newer baculovirus systems have modifications that permit the sole survival of the recombined viruses. The viruses are secreted into the culture medium and can be stored for long periods (up to 6 months at 4°C, longer at

−70°C). The formation of these virus particles is essential because the infected insect cells die after a while. New antibody-producing cells can then be generated at any time with the viruses. Large amounts of recombinant antibody fragments are formed with the help of the insect promoters, which can be secreted into the medium by fusion to a eukaryotic signal sequence.

Initially, a double infection with separate virus constructs for the light and heavy chain was used to be able to yield the gene for a complete immunoglobulin molecule in insect cells (Hasemann and Capra, 1990). Subsequently, a variety of practical improvements have been performed. One improvement represents the simultaneous recombination of both chains (zu Putlitz et al., 1990). Cassette systems enable the quick cloning of different recombinant antibody fragments (Poul et al., 1995). Nowadays, various baculovirus transfer vector combinations are commercially available from a wide range of companies. A more simple identification of successfully recombined viruses is possible with selection markers. Recently, vectors are also available (e.g., vEHuni) that allow direct cloning into the virus genome without the detour through a transfection vector. Optimized cell lines (e.g., "High Five" from *Trichoplasia ni*) with higher production rates are also available.

High yield (many mg/ml) cultures can be achieved (Holvoet et al., 1991; Laroche et al., 1991). A variety of different complete antibodies and recombinant antibody fragments have meanwhile been produced with the help of the baculovirus system. Examples include scFv monomers (Kretzschmar et al., 1996), mouse IgG (Nesbit et al., 1992), human-mouse chimeras (Hu et al., 1995), human IgA molecules (Carayannopoulos et al., 1994), or the Fab fragments of an IgM antibody (Abrams et al., 1994). Bifunctional proteins from recombinant antibody fragments and heterologous regions have also been expressed successfully, for example, a chorionic gonadotropin-IgG-Fc fusion (Johnson et al., 1995) or a scFv-IL2 fusion protein (Bei et al., 1995).

Baculovirus expression has even been used for the mutation analysis and screening of a gene library from recombinant antibody fragments (Potter et al., 1994; Ward et al., 1995)

A variety of different insect cells can be infected with baculovirus constructs. Baculoviruses (*Bombyx mori nuclear polyhedrosis virus*), which expressed both chains of a complete IgG2A molecule controlled by two independent polyhedrin promoters, have been successfully used to infect silkworm larvae. After 7 days 800 mg/l of recombinant antibody could be obtained from the hemolymph of the larvae (Reis et al., 1992).

The coexpression of a chaperone (BiP) could increase the amount of intracellular IgG formed, but not the amount of functional secreted product (Hsu et al., 1994). As already observed in *E. coli*, the addition of a single helper factor appears insufficient to imitate a plasma cell completely, in the complex processes during immunoglobulin folding in the endoplasmic reticulum. Expression in baculovirus however, is still one of the most widely used methods for the eukaryotic production of recombinant antibody fragments.

4.3.5 PRODUCTION OF RECOMBINANT ANTIBODY FRAGMENTS IN PLANTS

The production of recombinant antibody fragments in higher plants is an arduous process due to the long generation times and the complicated transformation procedure. The compensation however, is the potential to produce recombinant antibody fragments agriculturally. This production method, measured in terms of biomass, is doubtless cheaper than every other method that requires special nutritional media or laboratory methods. Therefore, the choice of this production method is reasonable when large amounts of recombinant antibody fragments are needed.

The plant used up to now for the production of recombinant antibody fragments is tobacco (*Nicotiana tabacum*). After genomic integration, plants could be obtained in which a heavy immunoglobulin chain constituted up to 1% of the soluble protein (Benvenuto et al., 1991). Usually, however, complete immunoglobulin chains were not produced, rather scFv fragments (Bruyns et al., 1996). Through the addition of a signal sequence, even secretion into the interstitial space between the plant cells was successful, such that the antibodies could be simply washed out from the leaves (Firek et al., 1993; Schouten et al., 1996).

Plant cell cultures were also used for the production of recombinant antibody fragments (Firek et al., 1993). It is certain that better methods are available, however, for production in eukaryotic suspension cultures. Therefore, this method might rather serve as a tool for quickly testing the antibody production during the generation of transgenic plants.

4.3.6 PRODUCTION OF RECOMBINANT ANTIBODY FRAGMENTS IN FUNGI

4.3.6.1 Production in Yeast

The single-celled yeast can be cultivated similarly to bacteria, in simple medium, in shaking cultures or fermenters. Their relatively fast growth also resembles bacteria but they present the advantages of a eukaryotic production and secretion apparatus. Their genetics are well investigated, and methods are established for the generation of transgenic yeast cells and the production of heterologous proteins. Therefore, their abilities have also been exploited, meanwhile, for the production of recombinant antibodies. The beer yeast, *Saccharomyces cerevisiae*, is the most frequently used. IgG and IgM molecules as well Fab fragments against various antigens have been produced in this yeast (Edqvist et al., 1991). Yields of up to 0.1% of the total protein have been achieved with vectors that lead to intracellular expression. In this case, however, only a small amount of the protein was functional (Bowdish et al., 1991). A secretion vector was also inserted into *Saccharomyces cerevisiae* that uses the phosphoglycerate kinase promoter and the invertase signal sequence. Active mouse–human chimeric antibodies could be obtained from the culture medium in this way. They were not correctly glycosylated, however, since they were able to mediate antibody-dependent cellular cytotoxicity but not to stimulate the complementary activity (Horwitz et al., 1988). The suitability of other yeast was also investigated for the production of recombinant antibodies. A *single-chain* antibody against fluorescein could be obtained from *Schizisaccharomyces pombe* (Davis et al., 1991), and various recombinant *single-chain* antibodies were secreted with high yields from *Pichia pastoris*. In this way, up to 100 mg/l of a functional, *single-chain* antibody, against human leukemia inhibitory factor, could be obtained from the culture medium of a simple shaking culture in the laboratory (Ridder et al., 1995b). This system can now be obtained commercially. In one case, it was discovered that, also in *Pichia*, the ordering of the V regions influences the yield. Of the two VH-linker-VL and the VL-linker-VH constructs, only the latter was produced (Luo et al., 1995). This study also proved that Fv fragments, stabilized through an artificially inserted disulfide bridge at the VH–VL interface (see also Section 2.4.10), could be successfully produced in *Pichia*.

4.3.6.2 Production in the Fungus *Trichoderma reesei*

Relatively high yields (1 mg/ml) of a recombinant Fab antibody fragment could be obtained from the culture medium of the filamentous fungus *Trichoderma reesei*. These fungi can be cultivated in a similarly uncomplicated way as yeast cells. The transformation procedure is somewhat more arduous, however. The yield could be increased to 150 mg/ml in a fermenter culture through the genetic fusion to the enzyme cellobiohydrolase I, which is produced in large amounts by the fungi and constitutes up to 50% of the total secreted protein in wild-type fungal cultures. The heterologous fusion portion was then split out from the culture medium by an uncharacterized protease, which could be coenriched by purification using ion exchange chromatography. Unfortunately, this promising system has been tested with only one recombinant antibody, so that statements about its general usefulness are not possible (Nyyssonen et al., 1993; Keranen and Penttila, 1995).

4.3.7 PRODUCTION IN CELL-FREE SYSTEMS

Expression in cell extracts is available as an alternative when a recombinant antibody fragment cannot be produced in a known system when, for example in the case of fusion to an extremely cytoxic protein to form an immunotoxin. Examples include fusions of an scFv fragment to the toxic regions of diphtheria toxin or *Pseudomonas* exotoxin A that were translated *in vitro* in a rabbit reticulocyte extract (Nicholls et al., 1993). The attainable yields are not suitable for applications outside the laboratory setting. This system also reaches its limits when used for the production of toxin fusions that impair ribosomal functions and thus, also inhibit synthesis in this *in vitro* system. Completely synthetic methods, such as peptide synthesis, are currently not yet able to manufacture polypeptides of the required lengths. Further development of peptide chemistry and automation, in combination with *in vitro* folding techniques, could make this approach gain importance in the future.

4.4 Purification of Recombinant Antibodies and Antibody Fragments

4.4.1 PHYSICAL SEPARATION METHODS ARE THE FIRST STEPS IN EVERY ANTIBODY PURIFICATION

The first step in purifying recombinant antibody fragments is to obtain the relevant fraction from the culture. In *E. coli* or eukaryotic secretion systems, this is achieved by pelleting the cells in a centrifuge. The medium can be freed of low molecular weight components by ultrafiltration and/or be concentrated. In instances of intracellular expression or secretion into the *E. coli* periplasma, cell disruption is required. A variety of different protocols are available, from mechanical homogenization to enzymatic lysis of the cell wall. This first, physical purification step often already allows a significant enrichment of the desired product. The subsequent enrichment steps are usually carried out in the form of column chromatography.

Naturally, the vast choice of different chromatographic purification protocols for proteins is also available for recombinant antibody fragments. Most frequently used are ion exchange chromatography and size exclusion chromatography. Another separation principle that can be used to purify recombinant antibody fragments is thiophilic adsorption chromatography (Schulze et al., 1994). With this method, scFv fragments from *E. coli* extracts could be so strongly concentrated that purification to homogeneity only required one more step.

4.4.2 AFFINITY CHROMATOGRAPHY: THE KEY TO EFFICIENT PURIFICATION OF RECOMBINANT PROTEINS

All these methods are usually combined with other purification procedures in several steps. Thus, the achievable concentration factors in ion exchange chromatography or size exclusion chromatography are limited by the relatively crude classification according to net charge or Stoke's radius. The use of specific binding as a separation technique results in substantially improved enrichments. These concentration methods are collectively termed *affinity chromatography*. For most recombinantly produced antibody fragments, a two-step purification strategy has proved sufficient for the isolation of amply purified material from cell extracts or cell culture media. This comprises a combination of affinity chromatography with a subsequent column chromatography. In the case of *E. coli* expression of scFv fragments, this second step is often size exclusion chromatography that serves to separate aggregates and dimers from monomers (e.g., Whitlow et al., 1993; Kipriyanov et al., 1994).

Affinity chromatography methods have thus largely dominated as the main purification step for recombinant antibodies. Within these, two groups of purification methods exist. One group can be characterized as *antigen-specific methods* and is based on the desired function of the recombinant antibody fragment itself: the antigen recognition. By contrast, the second group uses the epitope properties of the antibody chains to achieve specific binding to the column material. These *antibody-specific methods* are not dependent on the antigen specificity. This can only be achieved in instances where a respective binding region is still a component of the recombinant protein. Thus, the Fc portions or the constant regions of Fab' fragments are required for effective chromatography with protein A or G (for exceptions see below). When such interaction domains are not available, as is the case with scFv fragments, the genetic fusion of recombinant antibodies to small peptide fragments called *tags* is used. These *tags* can mediate specific binding to column material. Examples for both antigen- and antibody-specific methods will be given in the following Sections.

4.4.3 AFFINITY CHROMATOGRAPHIC PURIFICATION WITH THE HELP OF THE BINDING PROPERTIES OF THE ANTIBODY PORTION

4.4.3.1 Purification Through Antigen Binding

Binding to the antigen by an antibody usually occurs with very high specificity and an affinity in the submicromolar range, because it has been optimized to do this by evolution. So, theoretically, from a cell extract from *E. coli* or from culture medium only the antibody fragments can bind to the antigen column. The enrichment factors that can be achieved are therefore significant, but frequently, elution in a pH range of below 3 is needed because of the very high affinity. This can already lead to denaturation and the subsequent loss of active antibodies for some recombinant antibodies, especially Fv derivatives without the portion of the stabilizing constant chains. The conditions for the antigen affinity chromatography must be therefore determined for each antigen–antibody pair separately. Nevertheless, this method is an attractive alternative to the universal purification methods in cases where sufficient antigen is available. A single-chain Fv fragment, against the plant enzyme phytochrome from transgenic tobacco plants, could be enriched to near homogeneity in one step by this method (Owen et al., 1992). Similarly, an immunotoxin against the human IL2 receptor could be obtained in one step, from *in vitro* refolded material from *E. coli* inclusion bodies (Spence et al., 1993). Another example is the purification of an anti-erbB 2 scFv fragment from myeloma cell culture medium on erbB 2 Sepharose (Dorai et al., 1994).

4.4.3.2 Purification With the Help of Antiidiotypic Antibodies

A special case is represented by the purification on antiidiotypic antibody columns. Here, it is not the native antigen that is immobilized on the separation column but an antibody that recognizes the antigen binding site (the idiotype) of the recombinant antibody to be purified (Ayala et al., 1992). This method is especially of use when there is not a sufficient amount of antigen available, or when it is not suitable for coupling to column material because of its structure. This applies to some integral membrane proteins that lose the antigen determinant through solubilization. Establishing a purification method based on antiidiotypic antibodies is only worthwhile in exceptional cases. The cost and effort of producing such idiotypic antibodies is certainly greater than any needed to establish one of the universal purification methods.

A further modification of the antigen-specific affinity chromatography is the use of antigen analogues (Anthony et al., 1992). When antigen analogues for an antibody are known, they can substitute the native antigen in purification. Ideally, analogues with lower binding affinities compared to the original antigen are used to allow the use of more gentle elution conditions. Analogues can also be advantageous when the natural ligand is too unstable for coupling to the column material, or does not possess the appropriate functional groups for chemical coupling.

4.4.3.3 Purification With Immunoglobulin-Binding Proteins

A wide range of immunoglobulin-binding molecules is available for the purification of antibodies. An obvious possibility is the use of antibodies against the immunoglobulin to be purified. For example, a chimeric Fab' fragment, comprising a human constant region and a murine Fv region against carcinoembryonic antigen (CEA) was purified with the help of antibodies against human kappa chains (Chester et al., 1994).

Bacterial immunoglobulin-binding molecules are more frequently used. These binding molecules have been developed particularly by bacteria that encounter the immune response. The binding molecules allow them to cover their surfaces with immunoglobin molecules, with which they camouflage themselves from the immune system. Four different bacterial binding molecules are used for antibody purification meanwhile: proteins A, G, L, and H.

Protein A is a 42 kDa surface protein from *Staphylococcus aureus*. Binding to immunoglobulins of many different species occurs through the Fc portion of the antibody. Only a few Fab' molecules are bound by protein A (Erntell et al., 1986), especially those with heavy chains of subgroup III (Sasso et al., 1991). Due to this restriction, protein A is usually used for the purification of complete IgG molecules or molecules that possess the Fc portion (e.g., miniantibodies consisting of scFv+Fc). It is not usually used for the purification of recombinant antibody fragments from *E. coli* (Kelley et al., 1992). Detection agents for immunoassays (fluorescent, enzyme or gold conjugates) of protein A are commercially available in various forms.

Protein G is a 30–35 kDa surface protein of *Streptococcus* strain G148. Protein G binds to a wide spectrum of complete antibodies. An overview is given in Table 4.5. One very useful property for the purification of recombinant antibody fragments from *E. coli* is the binding of protein G to Fab' fragments. A domain inside the protein, other than that which binds to the Fc portion, is responsible for this (Erntell et al., 1988). The two regions can be expressed separately and thus allow a separate purification of Fc portions (Goward et al., 1990). A further domain of the protein binds serum albumin. This disturbs the purification of recombinant antibody fragments from expression systems that require serum in the growth medium. Recombinant expression of a variant of protein G that does not possess this binding domain has meanwhile been performed successfully.

The binding of protein G to Fab' fragments is also dependent on the sequence of the antibody. Not all Fab' fragments bind to protein G, and when they do, the affinity can be very different. The differential binding ability to recombinant antibody fragments (without the Fc portion) can, however, be put to use in a differential purification scheme. Fab' fragments could be selectively separated from F(ab')$_2$ fragments from a mouse–human chimera of the antitumor antibody B72.3 from recombinant CHO cells (Proudfoot et al., 1992). The elution of the Fab' fragments was thus possible under very mild conditions at neutral pH. This must, of course, be tested for each individual case.

A large number of various antibodies were purified with the help of protein G, including recombinant chimeras and humanized antibodies (Carter et al., 1992; Kelly et al., 1992). Due to its frequent use, purification technology with the help of protein G is well established. Commercial column materials are available in several forms (Bill et al., 1995). Detection agents (fluorescent, enzyme or gold conjugates) are also commercially available in various forms. A protein G variant from *Streptococcus suis* capsular type 2 possesses a lower affinity to most Ig forms but binds extremely well to chicken immunoglobulins (Serhir et al., 1995). Only a few chicken antibodies have been recombinantly

Table 4.5   Binding Specificity of Protein A and Protein G

Type	Subclass	Binding to Protein A	Binding to Protein G
Man	IgG1	++++	++++
	IgG2	++++	++++
	IgG3	−	++++
	IgG4	++++	++++
Mouse	IgG1	+	++++
	IgG2a	++++	++++
	IgG2b	+++	+++
	IgG3	++	+++
Rat	IgG1	−	+
	IgG2a	−	++++
	IgG2b	−	++
	IgG2c	+	++
Rabbit		++++	+++
Guinea pig		++++	++
Sheep		+/−	++
Goat		−	++
Horse		++	++++
Pig		+++	+++
Cow		++	++++
Hamster		+	++
Chicken		−	+
Dog		+	+/−

(Compiled from Harlow and Lane (1988) and various authors as given in Section 4.4.3.3)

produced to date (see also Section 2.2.5.3), but the development of gene libraries and the simple rearing of these animals could bring about a stronger interest in this species in the future. The interaction of various antibody sequences with protein G can vary significantly. Therefore, the loading and elution conditions must be newly optimized for every recombinant antibody fragment, particularly in the use of the Fab' binding region.

Protein L, a 72 kDa protein from the cell surface of the anaerobic bacteria *Peptostreptococcus magnus*, binds with high affinities (1.5×10^9 M^{-1}) to kappa chains, but only weakly to lambda chains. Approximately 75% of the various antibodies are recognized by protein L (Akerstrom et al., 1989). Binding occurs at the variable region (Sohi et al., 1995). Not all the human kappa subgroups are recognized, however. Only the human kappa subgroups I and III are bound well. Contrastingly, the kappa subgroup II and all lambda subgroups are not (Nilson et al., 1992). Protein L also binds the kappa chains from the mouse, rabbit, rat, and a few primates (De Chateau et al., 1993). In the humanization of mouse antibodies, the framework regions can be chosen that enable a specific purification of the product with protein L. This worked for a mouse – human hybrid with a protein L -binding kappa subtype III chain (Nilson et al., 1993). Protein L is therefore also suitable for the purification of smaller recombinant antibody fragments such as scFvs or Fabs with kappa VL regions. Once again, each individual case must be tested for the existence of a binding kappa subgroup.

Protein H is a 42 kDa surface protein of the group A streptococci (strain AP1) and binds to immunoglobulins in a temperature-dependent fashion. The affinity constant of binding to human polyclonal IgG is 1.6×10^9 (Akesson et al., 1990). It especially binds human IgG1 to IgG4, human IgG Fc portions and rabbit IgG. Binding was not observed to IgG from the mouse, rat, cow, sheep, or goat, nor to human IgA, IgD, IgE, or IgM (Gomi et al., 1990). Binding can occur at 22°C and is abolished by warming to 37°C (Akerstrom et al., 1992). The strongly restricted species specificity limits the use of protein H in the purification of recombinant antibody fragments. Protein H may play a larger role in the future for the gentle purification of recombinant human antibody fragments because of its temperature-dependent binding.

A whole range of further bacterial immunoglobulin-binding molecules has been described, but not yet been thoroughly investigated for their use in the purification and detection of recombinant antibody fragments. New methods will surely arise in the future.

4.4.3.4 Several Types of scFv Fragments Can Also Be Purified With the Help of Immunoglobulin-Binding Molecules

Some bacterial binding molecules possess an affinity and specificity to Fv fragments that is sufficient for purification. An extensive study that investigated the interaction of 34 human, *single-chain* antibodies with various bacterial binding proteins showed that, as expected, not all scFv fragments are equally well suited to a corresponding purification (Akerstrom et al., 1994). Some scFv fragments bound to *Staphylococcus* protein A and *Peptostreptococcus* protein L but not to the streptococcal proteins G or H. Affinities up to 1.4×10^9 M^{-1} were achieved for binding to protein L, but only two of the 34 investigated scFv fragments bound at this strength. In these cases, protein L- or A- Sepharose could be used for purification directly from the *E. coli* culture medium. The binding to protein A was specific for sequences of the subgroup VH3 of the heavy chain in the group of scFv fragments investigated, but only half the antibodies with this VH region bound. Protein L, which binds to the VL region, was investigated for its reaction with members of the kappa 1, kappa 4, lambda 1, lambda 2, and lambda 3 subgroups. It reacted with all kappa 1 sequences, one of the lambda 2, and one of the lambda 3 regions. A sequence comparison of the investigated antibodies did not yield a clear consensus structure for binding. The contributing amino acid residues are apparently distributed over a large part of the framework regions.

4.4.4 AFFINITY CHROMATOGRAPHIC PURIFICATION WITH THE HELP OF A HETEROLOGOUS FUSION COMPONENT

Not only the recombinant antibody regions themselves, but also heterologous fusion components, or protein domains chemically coupled to the antibody fragments, can be employed for a specific enrichment. These methods are differentiated into two groups for practical reasons. In the first instance, a protein fragment is appended that serves to impart a new biochemical function to the molecule, that is, to the creation of a bifunctional molecule. These heterologous components are autonomous protein domains and often have their own ligands. Many examples are shown in Sections 3.2 and 3.3. Only a few cases are introduced here, in which the specific binding properties of these heterologous components have been exploited for purification.

In the other case, the heterologous fusion components are designed particularly for the purpose of purifying or detecting the construct. Therefore, an effort is made to make these protein components as small as possible. Most systems are based on small, linear, (unstructured) peptide extensions of about 10 amino acid residues. These are defined as *tags*.

4.4.4.1 Affinity Chromatographic Purification With the Help of the Binding Properties of a Heterologous Fusion Component

In general, the purification methods using larger heterologous fusion components represent special cases that are limited to particular constructs. They are available only when the heterologous fusion component binds to agents that can be obtained in large quantities and can be coupled to a column. The dye Cibacon Blue is used for the purification of some plant toxins. In the given example, a fusion protein from toxin and recombinant antibody was purified with this dye (Better et al., 1993, 1994). *Staphylococcus aureus* protein A domains, used to interact with other antibodies in fusion proteins, can also be used for purification. In this way, protein A::antiphytochrome single-chain Fv fusion proteins were successfully purified on IgG agarose (Gandecha et al., 1992).

The maltose-binding protein (MBP) was also employed to enrich recombinant antibody fragments. This protein binds specifically to the polysaccharide amylose. Thus, MBP fused Fv and scFv fragments were purified successfully on crosslinked amylose (Bregegere et al., 1994). This fusion to a rather large heterologous protein was exclusively used for the purpose of purification. Alternative methods, such as the use of shorter *tags* (see below) should usually be more advantageous in most cases.

Another example for purification by the binding of a heterologous fusion component has been demonstrated for scFv fusions with streptavidin. ScFv fusion proteins that contained a *core* streptavidin could be purified by affinity chromatography with analogues of biotin. In this case, the natural ligand, biotin, could not be used due to its extremely high affinity (a binding constant of roughly 10^{-14} M), which does not allow the elution of the fusion protein under native conditions. By contrast, the low-affinity biotin analogues, 2-iminobiotin and diaminobiotin, enabled the enrichment of the fusion protein. Here, a very gentle elution was conducted with either an excess of soluble analogue or biotin (Dübel et al., 1995), or through a lowering of the pH. The latter, however, lead to a loss of correctly folded scFv fragments (Kipriyanov et al., 1995b).

4.4.4.2 Purification With the Help of *tags*

Short peptides, which allow an affinity chromatographic purification of recombinant antibody fragments through specific binding to another molecule, are called *tags*. They are usually appended to the amino terminus or the carboxy terminus of recombinant antibody fragments by genetic fusion. The carboxy terminus of one of the variable domains is usually chosen as the fusion point because the C termini of the variable domains are farthest away from the antigen-binding site of the antibody. There are also a few *tags* inserted as internal sequences. For example, the Yol1/34 epitope (..EEGEFSEAR..) is an octapeptide from alpha tubulin (Breiting and Little, 1986) built into the peptide linker of scFv fragments between the VH and the VL region (Breitling et al., 1991).

4.4.4.3 The His *tag* Allows Affinity Chromatography on Immobilized Metals (IMAC)

Oligohistidine peptides can bind nickel, copper, or zinc ions with sufficient affinity. When these divalent cations are bound to immobilized chelates, they can be employed for a chromatographic enrichment of proteins that carry a *tag* of 3–6 histidines (see overview in Sulkowski, 1985). The binding mechanism is illustrated in Figure 4.3.

Elution can be done at nearly neutral pH with an excess of imidazole, which can later be removed by dialysis. Thus, an elution is available that is milder than that for most other *tags*. This method, *immobilized metal affinity chromato-graphy* (IMAC) or *metal chelate affinity chromatography* (MCAC) represents probably the most widely used purification step for recombinant antibody fragments from *E. coli* and other nonmammalian expression systems. Its main advantages are the robust nature of the column and the mild elution conditions. The binding is not affected by denaturing agents such as urea and thus, a purifi-cation of scFv fragments in a denatured state is possible before an *in vitro* folding (Burks and Iverson, 1995; Kipriyanov et al., 1995a). This compensates

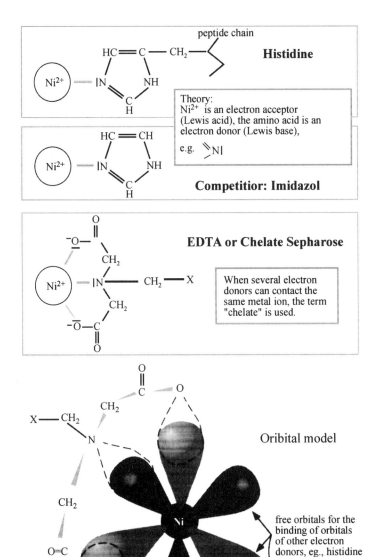

Fig. 4.3. The binding theory of IMAC: orbital model for the binding of Mg, Cu, or Zn to a chelate.

for one of the disadvantages of the His *tag*, its low specificity. A large number of proteins contain metal-binding sites (e.g., the zinc finger proteins) and therefore, they can equally bind to immobilized nickel or zinc ions, and limit the degree of enrichment. The metal-binding sites of these proteins must be maintained in the correct secondary/tertiary structure and thus, chromatography in the presence of denaturing agents also allows a separation from these proteins. Additionally, a His_6 *tag* can bind to several ions, thus achieving a higher binding avidity. The high concentration of imidazole that is necessary for elution (typically greater than 200 mmol/l) enables a differential elution of the impurities at lower concentrations of imidazole. To avoid nonspecific binding due to ion exchange effects, the separation is usually performed at high ionic strength. Typically, 1 M NaCl but also 0.5 M K_2SO_4 have been successfully employed.

IMAC had been used previously for the enrichment of various fusion proteins from *E. coli* and quickly became the standard method for the purification of scFv fragments (Skerra et al., 1991; Dübel et al., 1992) and Fab fragments (Skerra, 1994).

A change in the stoichiometric relationship between VH to VL was observed in IMAC purification of Fv fragments, in which both chains carried a hexahistidine *tag*. This effect could be prevented when the zwitterion betaine, a very soluble osmolyte comprising a negatively charged carboxyl group and a positively charged quaternary amino group, was used to replace the normal salt (Essen and Skerra, 1993).

A large number of various recombinant antibodies (Ayala et al., 1995; Molloy et al., 1995), their fusion proteins with heterologous effector components (Newton et al., 1994; Thielemans, 1995) and, among others, various scFv fragments obtained from IgM (Jahn et al., 1995; Rosso et al., 1996) could be purified with the help of IMAC. His-*tags* were also successfully used for the purification of scFv fragments from eukaryotic cell cultures (Dorai et al., 1994). The degree of enrichment can be strongly influenced by the choice of column material and elution conditions (Canaan-Haden et al., 1995). Empirically, column materials which complex the ion with two chelating arms (e.g., iminodiacetic acid resins) are advantageous for purification of proteins with shorter His tags (from 3-5 His residues), which were not optimally retained on materials with three chelating arms (e.g., NTA resins). For larger preparations, the optimization of these factors is recommended, depending on the starting material (*E. coli* periplasma/inclusion bodies, eukaryotic cell culture medium).

Not much is known about the effect of the *his tag* on the pharmacokinetic parameters of recombinant antibodies. However, the distribution within an organism of an anticarcinoembryonic antigen (CEA) scFv fragment has been investigated. It was discovered that the His *tag* did not alter the distribution in the tissue or the enrichment at the tumor (Casey et al., 1995).

A procedure analogous to the IMAC purification described above was used to purify a bispecific mouse–human hybrid antibody against CEA and indium benzyl EDTA with TSK-SP-5-PW ion exchange material (Beidler et al., 1991). This and similar constructs, which are to be used for radioimaging or radiotherapy *in vivo*, already carry a metal-binding region (in this case, a recombinant antibody fragment) as a fusion component. This metal-binding region serves to complex the radioisotope. Therefore, these proteins do not need a special His *tag* for the purification described.

The dialysis step can be omitted in quick tests in which IMAC-enriched recombinant antibody fragments are to be used. Instead of imidazole, they can be eluted with 100–200 mM EDTA. This elutes the scFv fragment together with the nickel ions. The column can equilibrated to low salt buffer before this step.

Besides speed, the omission of the dialysis provides a further advantage. The eluate sample can be stored for long periods due to the antimicrobial effect of nickel and EDTA (Dübel et al., 1995). ScFv fragments produced in this way can be directly used for immunoblots, ELISA or FACS.

Agents have recently become available that allow detection of the His *tag* in immunological tests, such as immunoblots or ELISA. Two different groups of agents have proved successful:

1. Monoclonal antibodies against the His hexapeptide. Various antibodies have been described. Those that recognize the peptide in different positions (at the carboxy terminus, the amino terminus, or even as an internal epitope) are to be preferred.
2. The spectrum of applications for enzyme chelate conjugates is even wider. There are now commercially available nickel-NTA enzyme conjugates that not only recognize *tags* containing six histidines in every possible arrangement, but also *tags* with fewer histidines. Their disadvantage is the omission of the amplification step created by the sandwich assembly of the antibody-dependent dye system. They are sufficient, however, for routine uses such as the detection of recombinant antibody fragments in bacterial colony blots, immunoblots, or in ELISA.

4.4.4.4 The FLAG Peptide System: An Antibody for Purification and Detection

The hydrophilic "FLAG" octapeptide DYKDDDDK (Boothe et al., 1988) was used for the detection and purification of a variety of recombinant expression products. It can be appended to the amino terminus as well as the carboxy terminus of recombinant antibody fragments.

The core epitope was narrowed down to a pentapeptide with the sequence YKXXD through the screening of a phage display library (Miceli et al., 1994). A partial sequence of the octapeptide of only four amino acid residues in length, DYKD, still bound with sufficient affinity to the anti-FLAG antibody (Knappik and Plückthun, 1994). It was established, however, that the following amino acid position also affected the binding affinity. The last amino acid of this minimal epitope is an aspartic acid residue. Therefore, the heterologous component of a recombinant antibody fragment can be reduced even to three amino acid residues in some cases because aspartic acid is the most frequent amino acid residue in position 1 of the VL region. This peptide is thus the shortest antibody epitope used for the recognition and purification of recombinant antibody fragments, to date. Apart from the FLAG peptide, only His *tags* allow a specific affinity chromatographic enrichment with only three additional amino acid residues.

The monoclonal antibody M1 recognizes the FLAG peptide and is dependent on the simultaneous binding of calcium ions. This property can be exploited when recombinant antibody fragments require mild elution conditions. Removal of calcium leads to a drastic reduction in the affinity and allows an elution without changes in pH (Hopp et al., 1996).

4.4.4.5 The c-*myc tag* (*myc*1-9E10 Epitope)

The peptide ..EEQKLISEEDL.. is the epitope of the monoclonal mouse antibody Myc1-9E10 (Evan et al., 1985) and part of the cellular, human, 62 kDa oncoprotein, *myc* (c-*myc*). This high specificity antibody shows few cross-reactions and little nonspecific binding when *E. coli* whole-cell extracts are used. This makes it especially valuable for the control of expression from crude cell extracts of *E. coli* or other expression systems. A variety of constructs and detection systems for recombinant antibody fragments have been fused to this peptide in various immunological detection systems (e.g., Ward et al., 1989; Dreher et al., 1991; Dübel et al., 1993; Kleymann et al., 1995; Kontermann et al., 1995).

The c-*myc tag* has not only been used for detection but also for the column chromatographic purification of immobilized antibodies. Here, the monoclonal antibody Myc1-9E10 was coupled to Sepharose. The elution occurred at pH 3.0, a range in which the recombinant antibody fragments are not yet seriously harmed (Froyen et al., 1993). Other specific options of coupling an anti-*tag* antibody for purification by affinity chromatography have been successfully employed. The Myc1-9E10 antibody was incubated with protein A Sepharose and then covalently crosslinked with dimethyl-pimelidate. ScFv antibodies against T-cell antigens could be successfully purified with this column (Popov et al., 1996). A similar approach, but without crosslinking the protein A to the Myc1-9E10 antibody, allowed the elution of bifunctional scFv fragment/Myc1-9E10 complexes. An analogous noncovalent method of producing bifunctional recombinant antibody fragments can be used to improve their binding ability through increased avidity (Gotter et al., 1994).

Recently, the scFv fragment of the Myc1-9E10 antibody has been made available (Fuchs et al., 1997).

4.4.4.6 The "Strep *tag*": A Biotin Analogue With Lower Affinity

Streptavidin is a protein from the gram-positive bacterium *Streptomyces avidinii* with functional similarity to chicken egg avidin. It comprises four identical 15 kDa subunits. A special feature is its extremely high affinity for biotin. It belongs to the strongest noncovalent bonds described with a binding constant of roughly 10^{-14} M. The "strep *tag*" is a synthetic peptide of nine amino acid residues (AWRHPQFGG), which binds to streptavidin with an affinity (2.7×10^4 M^{-1}) that is sufficient for purification by column chromatography (Schmidt et al., 1996). It uses the binding pocket for biotin, and can be employed for purification and detection of proteins by fusion to their carboxytermini. The peptide was isolated from a peptide gene library (see also Section 2.3.3) (Schmidt and Skerra, 1993). It allows both the purification by column chromatography of the corresponding fusion protein with streptavidin agarose, and also the detection of the fusion protein on immunoblots and in ELISAs with the help of a streptavidin enzyme conjugate. The degree of enrichment that can be obtained is often sufficient to enable a purification of recombinant antibody fragments in one step, because of its very specific binding. Various membrane proteins from *Paracoccus denitrificans* and *Halobacterium halobium* could be detected by electron microscopy using gold labeled streptavidin with Fv fragments purified in this way from *E. coli* (Kleymann et al., 1995). A disadvantage of the strep *tag* is that it only functions when fused to the carboxy terminus. The newer strep *tag* II has the sequence SNWSHPQFEK, and possesses a twofold lower affinity for streptavidin than the peptide described above. In contrast to the original peptide, the strep *tag* II also functions as a N-terminal fusion (Schmidt et al., 1996; Skerra, personal communication). This system has been further improved recently by engineering streptavidin to increase its affinity to *Strep tag* II by more than one order of magnitude compared with wild-type streptavidin by random mutagenesis of the amino acid residues 44-47 phage display (Voss and Skerra, 1997).

4.4.4.7 Choosing a Suitable *tag*

The choice of the *tag* sequences for a particular application is made according to the following criteria:

1. Highly specific binding should allow effective enrichment and the simple detection of the recombinant antibody fragment.
2. The affinity should not be too high so that mild elution conditions are possible during the purification.
3. The sequence should be as short as possible to minimize impairing the function of the recombinant antibody fragment.

These properties are offered by the strep *tags* in an ideal way. The His *tag* is currently more widely used, despite its lower specificity. Its advantage lies especially in the robust nature of the column material that can also be used under strongly denaturing conditions. When the addition of amino acid residues is feared potentially to disrupt the function of a recombinant antibody fragment, a *tag* that is as short as possible should be resorted to, such as the 3–4 amino acid residue long, improved, FLAG peptide. Alternatively, a cutting site for specific proteases can be incorporated between the antibody and the *tag* in some systems. This allows the heterologous sequence to be removed after the affinity chromatography or even for elution from the *tag*-bound column. The size of the *tag* is then no longer relevant. This scenario is only recommended for particular uses. In a carboxy terminal fusion, the *tag* is localized at the end of the antibody that is spatially opposite to the antigen binding site. Steric hindrance of antigen binding is therefore not to be expected. When used as a therapeutic in humans, the nonhuman sequence component can lead to an immune reaction against the recombinant antibody fragment and to the subsequent impairment of its function. Removal then improves the tolerance and efficacy of such a therapeutical agent.

The identification of a peptide sequence against which an IgG antibody present in the blood of all humans is directed (e.g., a sequence from *E. coli*), would be of interest. Virtually complete IgGs would then result after the injection of a Fv fragment with this sequence.

4.4.5 SPECIAL CASE HUMAN THERAPEUTIC AGENTS: REMOVAL OF BACTERIAL ENDOTOXINS

Antibody fragments produced in *E. coli* could be directly used in patients for example, in the form of immunotoxins for fighting tumors or for their detection by radioimaging. However, *E. coli* culture media often contain large amounts of lipopolysaccharides (LPS) from the outer cell membrane of the bacteria that can generate severe fever in humans. Therefore, these endotoxins must be quantitatively removed from the recombinant antibody fraction before administration to the patient. A whole range of methods ensures this removal.

High-affinity binding of endotoxins to the cationic antibiotic polymyxin had been observed. Affinity chromatography over polymyxin sepharose allowed the removal of LPS even from largely impure samples (Issekutz, 1983). Corresponding column materials are also offered commercially (Talmadge and Siebert, 1989). Immobilized histamine was also used for the removal of endotoxins (Minobe et al., 1983). More unspecific methods, such as gel filtration, are equally useable for the removal of high molecular weight endotoxins (Better and Gavit, 1997). A separate step to remove LPS is usually no longer needed in the purification of recombinant antibody fragments when an affinity chromatography step is used.

4.4.6 STORAGE OF PURIFIED RECOMBINANT ANTIBODIES

The long-term storage of some forms of recombinant antibody fragments represents a substantial problem. The production of complete IgG molecules and Fab or F(ab')$_2$ fragments presents the fewest difficulties. Antibodies are the defense system of the body, and constructed in a robust form. A durability of many years at 4°C is not uncommon. The addition of antibacterial agents, such as thimerosal (sodium ethyl mercury thiosalicylate) or sodium azide, is recommended in every case. However, for long-term storage, the antibodies should be frozen at −70°C in aliquots. Care must be taken that the solutions are not too dilute when frozen (not less than roughly 0.1 g/l total protein). The *single-chain* fragments again are a special case because they aggregate at high protein concentrations. This aggregation can be explained by two reasons. First, a portion of the surface of Fv fragments comprises an area that is not accessible to the surrounding solution in the intact immunoglobulin molecule. Therefore, it can mediate increased nonspecific adherence. Second, the low affinity of the binding of the VL to the VH enables binding of oligomers and finally aggregates (see Section 2.4.9). The constant domains of Fab fragments assist the stability of the correct dimers and thus, this effect is hardly noticeable here. A solution to this problem in the use of Fv fragments is a stabilization by a disulfide bridge at the VL-VH interface instead of a peptide linker (see Section 2.4.10).

Some scFv fragments have proved to be very stable and could be stored in their functional form for more than one year at 4°C without protective protein. The addition of a protective protein (usually BSA) in high concentrations (10–20 mg/ml) is recommended for less stable scFv fragments, when this is not disruptive in subsequent applications. The samples should then be stored in aliquots at temperatures of −70°C to −80°C. When the addition of a protective protein is not possible, recombinant antibody fragments can be stored similarly to enzymes after the addition of freeze protection agents such as glycerin, at −20°C.

Overall, repeated freezing and thawing should be avoided (Kortt et al., 1994), as this results in loss through aggregation, even in native IgG molecules, because the formation of ice crystals causes damage to the hydration coat of the proteins.

References

Abrams C, Deng YJ, Steiner BO, Toole T, Shattil SJ (1994) Determinants of specificity of a baculovirus-expressed antibody Fab fragment that binds selectively to the activated form of integn alpha IIb beta 3. *J Biol Chem* **269**:18781–18788.

Adams GP, McCartney JE, Tai MS, Oppermann H, Huston JS, Stafford WF, Bookman MA, Fand I, Houston LL, Weiner LM (1993) Highly specific *in vivo* tumor targeting by monovalent and divalent forms of 741F8 anti-c-*erb*-B-2 single-chain Fv. *Cancer Res* **53**:4026–4034.

Akerstrom B, Bjorck L (1989) Protein L: an immunoglobulin light chain-binding bacterial protein. Characterization of binding and physico-chemical properties. *J Biol Chem* **264**:19740–19746.

Akerstrom M, Lindahl G, Bjorck L, Lindqvist A (1992) Protein Arp and protein H from group A streptococci. Ig binding dimerization are regulated by temperature. *J Immunol* **148**:3238–3243.

Akerstrom B, Nilson BH, Hoogenboom HR, Bjorck L (1994) On the interaction between single chain Fv antibodies and bacterial immunoglobulin-binding proteins. *J Immunol Methods* **177**:151–163.

Akesson P, Cooney I, Kishimoto F, Bjorck L (1990) Protein H-a novel IgG binding bacterial protein. *Mol Immunol* **27**:523–531.

Ames RS, Tornetta MA, Deen K, Jones CS, Swift AM, Ganguly S (1995) Conversion of murine Fabs isolated from a combinatorial phage display library to full length immunoglobulins. *J Immunol Methods* **184**:177–186.

Anand NN, Mandal S, MacKenzie CR, Sadowska J, Sigurskjold B, Young NM, Bundle DR, Narang SA (1991) Bacterial expression and secretion of various single-chain Fv genes encoding proteins specific for a Salmonella sero type B O-antigen. *J Biol Chem* **266**:21874–21879.

Anthony J, Near R, Wong SL, Iida E, Ernst E, Wittekind M, Haber E (1992) Ng, SC Production of stable anti-digoxin Fv in *Escherichia coli*. *Mol Immunol* **29**:1237–1247.

Ayala M, Duenas M, Santos A, Vazquez J, Menendez A, Silva A, Gavilondo JV (1992) Bacterial single-chain antibody fragments, specific for carcinoembryonic antigen. *Biotechniques* **13**:790–799.

Ayala M, Balint RF, Fernandez de Cossio L, Canaan-Haden JW, Larrick JW, Gavilondo JV (1995) Variable region sequence modulates periplasmic export of a single-chain FV antibody fragment in *Escherichia coli*. *Biotechniques* **18**:832, 835–838, 840–842.

Barry MM, Lee JS (1993) Cloning and expression of an autoimmune DNA-binding single chain FV: only the heavy chain is required for binding. *Mol Immunol* **30**:833–840.

Bashford CL, Harris DA (1988) Spectrophotometry and Spectrofluorometry. IRL Press, Oxford, UK.

Beil R, Schiom J, Kashmiri SV (1995) Baculovirus expression of a functional single-chain immunoglobulin and its IL-2 fusion protein. *J immunol Methods* **186**:245–255.

Beidler DE, Johnson MJ, Unger BW, Phelps JL, Jue RA (1991) Purification and characterization of a chimeric bifunctional antibody specific for human carcinoembryonic antigen and indium-benzyl-EDTA. *Protein Exp Purif* **2**:76–82.

Bender E, Woof JM, Atkin JD, Barker MD, Bebbington CR, Burton DR (1993) Recombinant human antibodies: linkage of an Fab fragment from a combinatorial library to an Fc fragment for expression in mammalian cell culture. *Hum Antibodies Hybridomas* **4**:74–79.

Benvenuto E, Ordas RJ, Tavazza R, Anoora G, Biocca S, Cattaneo A, Galeffi P (1991) 'Phytoantibodies': a general vector for the expression of immunoglobulin domains in transgenic plants. *Plant Mol Biol* **17**:865–874.

Better M, Gavit P (1997) Production of antibody domains in prokaryotes. Antibody Therapeutics. CRC Press, Orlando, FL.

Better M, Cheng CP, Robinson RR, Horowitz AH (1988) *Escherichia coli* secretion of an active chimeric antibody fragment. *Science* **240**:1041–1043.

Better M, Berhard SL, Lei SP, Fishwild DM, Lane JA, Carroll SF, Horwitz AH (1993) Potent anti-CD4 ricin A chain immunoconjugates from bacterially produced Fab' F(ab')2. *Proc Natl Acad Sci USA* **90**:457–461.

Better M, Berhard SL, Fishwild DM, Nolan PA, Bauer RJ, Kung AH, Carroll SF (1994) Gelonin analogs with engineered cysteine residues form antibody immunoconjugates with unique properties. *J Biol Chem* **269**:9644–9650.

Bill E, Lutz U, Karlsson BM, Sparrman M, Allgaier H (1995) Optimization of protein G chromatography for biopharmaceutical monoclonal antibodies. *J Mol Recognit* **8**:90–94.

Booth RJ, Grandison PM, Prestidge RL, Watson JD (1988) The use of a 'universal' yeast expression vector to produce an antigenic protein of *Mycobacterium leprae*. *Immunol Lett* **19**:65–69.

Bowdish K, Tang Y, Hicks JB, Hilvert D (1991) Yeast expression of a catalytic antibody with chorismate mutase activity. *J Biol Chem* **266**:11901–11908.

Bregegere F, Schwartz J, Bedouelle H (1994) Bifunctional hybrids between the variable domains of an immunoglobulin and the maltose-binding protein of *Escherichia coli*: production, purification and antigen binding. *Protein Eng* **7**:271–280.

Breitling F, Little M (1986) Carboxy-terminal regions on the surface of tubulin and microtubules: epitope locations of YOL1/34, DM1A and DM1B. *J Mol Biol* **189**:367–370.

Breitling F, Dübel S, Seehaus T, Klewinghaus I, Little M (1991) A surface expression vector for antibody screening. *Gene* **104**:147–153.

Brigido MM, Polymenis M, Stollar BD (1993) Role of mouse VH10 and VL gene segments in the specific binding of antibody to Z-DNA, analyzed with recombinant single chain Fv molecules. *J Immunol* **150**:469–479.

Brinkmann U, Reiter Y, Jung SH, Lee B, Pastan I (1993) A recombinant immunotoxin containing a disulfide-stabilized Fv fragment. *Proc Natl Acad Sci USA* **90**:7538–7542.

Brocker T, Karjalainen K (1995) Signals through T-cell receptor-zeta chain alone are insufficient to prime resting T-lymphocytes. *J Exp Med* **181**:1653–1659.

Brocks B, Rode HJ, Geriach E, Dübel S, Little M, Pfizenmaier K, Moosmayer D (1997) A TNF receptor antagonistic scFv, which is refractory to secretion in mammalian cells, is expressed as a soluble mono- and bivalent scFv derivative in insect cells using cassette baculovirus vectors. Immunotechnologhy. **3**:173–184.

Bruyns AM, De Jaeger G, De Neve M, De Wilde C, Van Montagu M, Depicker A (1996) Bacterial and plant-produced scFv proteins have similar antigen-binding properties. *FEBS Lett* **386**:5–10.

Buchner J, Rudolf R (1991) Renatuaration, purification and characterization of recombinant antibody fragments produced in *E. coli*. *Biotechnology* **9**:157–162.

Buchner J, Pastan I, Brinkmann U (1992a) A method for increasing the yield of properly folded recombinant fusion proteins: single-chain immuntoxins from renaturation of bacterial inclusion bodies. *Anal Biochem* **205**:263–270.

Buchner J, Brinkmann U, Pastan I (1992b) Renaturation of a single-chain immuntoxin facilitated by chaperones and protein disulfide isomerase. *Biotechnology NY* **10**:682–685.

Buchsbaum DJ (1995) Experimental approachs to increase radiolabeled antibody localization in tumors. *Cancer Res* **55**(23 Suppl):5729s–5732s.

Burks EA, Iverson BL (1995) Rapid, high-yield recovery of a recombinant digoxin binding single-chain Fv from *Escherichia coli*. *Biotechnol Prog* **11**:112–114.

Cabilly S, Riggs AD, Pande H, Shively JE, Holmes WE, Rey M, Perry LJ, Wetzel R, Heyneker HL (1984) Generation of antibody activity from immunoglobulin polypeptide chains produced in *Escherichia coli*. *Proc Natl Acad Sci USA* **81**:3273–3277.

Canaan Haden L, Ayala M, Fernandez-de-Cossio ME, Pedroso I, Rodes L, Gavilondo JV (1995) Purification and application of a single-chain Fv antibody fragment specific to hepatitis B virus surface antigen. *Biotechniques* **19**:606–608.

Carayannopoulos L, Max EE, Capra JD (1994) Recombinant human IgA expressed in insect cells. *Proc Natl Acad Sci USA* **91**:8348–8352.

Carter P, Kelley RF, Rodriguez ML, Snedecor B, Covarrubias M, Velligan MD, Wong WLT, Rowland AM, Kotts CE, Carver ME, Yang M, Bourell JH, Shepard HM, Henner D (1992) High level *E. coli* expression and production of a bivalent humanized antibody fragment. *Bio/Technology* **10**:163–167.

Casey JL, Keep PA, Chester KA, Robson L, Hawkins RE, Begent RH (1995) Purification of bacterially expressed single-chain Fv antibodies for clinical applications using metal chelate chromatography. *J Immunol Methods* **179**:105–116.

Chen C, Martin TM, Stavens S, Rittenberg MB (1994) Defective secretion of an immunoglobulin caused by mutations in the heavy chain complementarity determining region 2. *J Exp Med* **180**:577–586.

Chester KA, Robson L, Keep PA, Pedley RB, Boden JA, Boxer GM, Hawkins RE, Begent RH (1994) Production and tumour-binding characterization of a chimeric anti-CEA Fab expressed in *Escherichia coli*. *J Cancer* **57**:67–72.

Chothia C. Lesk AM (1987) Canonical structures for the hypervariable regions of immunoglobulins. *J Mol Biol* **196**:901–917.

Ciric B, Radulovic M, Dimitrijevic LJ, Jankov RM (1995) Effect of valency on binding properties of the antihuman IgM monoclonal antibody 202. *Hybridoma* **14**:537–544.

Colcher D, Bird R, Roselli M, Hardman KD, Johnson S, Pope S, Dodd SW, Pantoliano MW, Milenic DE, Schlom J (1990) *In vivo* tumor targeting of a recombinant single-chain antigen-binding protein. *J Natl Cancer Inst* **82**:1191–1197.

Conrad U, Becker K, Ziegner M, Walter G (1991) Immunoglobulin VH and VK genes of the BALB/c anti-foot-and-mouth disease virus (O1) VP1 response: cloning, characterization and transgenic mice. *Mol Immunol* **28**:1201–1209.

Davis GT, Bedzyk WD, Voss EW, Jacobs TW (1991) Single chain antibody (SCA) encoding genes: one-step construction and expression in eukaryotic cells. *Biotechnology NY* **9**:165–169.

De Chateau M, Nilson BH, Erntell M, Myhre E, Magnusson CG, Akerstrom B, Bjorck L (1993) On the interaction between protein L and immunoglobulins of various mammalian species. *Scand J Immunol* **37**:399–405.

Deng SJ, MacKenzie CR, Sadowska J, Michniewicz J, Young NM, Bundle DR, Narang SA (1994) Selection of antibody single-chain variable fragments with improved carbohydrate binding by phage display. *J Biol Chem* **269**:9533–9538.

Deyev SM, Lieber A, Radko BV, Polanovsky OL (1993) Production of recombinant antibodies in lymphoid and non-lymphoid cells. *FEBS Lett* **330**:111–113.

Dorai H, McCartney JE, Hudziak RM, Tai MS, Laminet AA, Houston LL, Huston JS, Oppermann H (1994) Mammalian cell expression of single-chain Fv (sFv) antibody proteins and their C-terminal fusions with interleukin-2 and other effector domains. *Biotechnology NY* **12**:890–897.

Dreher ML, Gherardi E, Skerra A, Milstein C (1991) Colony assays for antibody fragments expressed in bacteria. *J Immunol Methods* **139**:197–205.

Dübel S, Breitling F, Klewinghaus I, Little M (1992) Regulated secretion and purification of recombinant antibodies in *E. coli*. *Cell Biophys* **21**:69–80.

Dübel S, Breitling F, Fuchs P, Klewinghaus I, Little M (1993) A family of vectors for surface display and production of antibodies. *Gene* **128**:97–101.

Dübel S, Breitling F, Kontermann R, Schmidt T, Skerra A, Little M (1995) Bifunctional and multimeric complexes of streptavidin fused to single-chain antibodies (scFv). *J Immunol Methods* **178**:201–209.

Duenas M, Vazquez J, Ayala M, Soderlind E, Ohlin M, Perez L, Borrebaeck CA, Gavilondo JV (1994) Intra- and extracellular expression of an scFv antibody fragment in *E coli*: effect of bacterial strains and pathway engineering using GroES/L chaperonins. *Biotechniques* **16**:476–477, 480–483.

Duenas M, Ayala M, Vazquez J, Ohlin M, Soderlind E, Borrebaeck CA, Gavilondo JV (1995) A point mutation in a murine immunoglobulin V-region strongly influences the antibody yield in *Escherichia coli*. *Gene* **158**:61–66.

Edqvist J, Keranen S, Penttila M, Straby KB, Knowles JK (1991) Production of functional IgM Fab fragments by *Saccharomyces cerevisia*. *J Biotechnol* **20**:291–300.

Erntell M, Myhre EB, Kronvall G (1986) Non-Immune F(ab')2-and Fc-mediated interactions of mammalian immunoglobulins with *S aureus* and group C and G streptococci. *Acta Pathol Microbiol Immunol Scand* **94**:377–383.

Erntell M, Myhre EB, Sjobring U, Bjorck L (1988) Streptococcal protein G has affinity for both Fab- and Fc-fragments of human IgG. *Mol Immuno* **25**:121–126.

Essen LO, Skerra A (1993) Single-step purification of a bacterially expressed antibody Fv fragment by immobilized metal affinity chromatography in the presence of betaine. *J Chromatogr* A **657**:55–61.

Evan GI, Lewis GK, Ramsay G, Bishop M (1985) Isolation of monoclonal antibodies specific for human c-myc proto-oncogene poroduct. *Mol Cell Biol* **5**:3610–3616.

Evans MJ, Rollins SA, Wolff DW, Norin AJ, Rother RP, Therrien DM, Grijalva GA, Mueller JP, Nye SH, Squinto SP, Wilkins JA (1995) *In vitro* and *in vivo* inhibition of complement activity by a single-chain Fv fragment recognizing human C5. *Mol Immunol* **32**:1183–1195.

Firek S, Draper J, Owen MR, Gandecha A, Cockburn B, Whitelam GC (1993) Secretion of a functional single-chain Fv protein in transgenic tobacco plants and cell suspension culture. *Plant Mol Biol* **23**:861–879.

Friguet B, Chaffotte AF, Djavadi-Ohanianec LD, Goldberg ME (1985) Measurements of the true affinity constant in solution of antigen – antibody complexes by enzyme linked immunosorbent assay. *J Immunol Methods* **77**:305–319.

Froyen G, Ronsse I, Billiau A (1993) Bacterial expression of a single-chain antibody fragment (SCFV) that neutralizes the biological activity of human interferon-gamma. *Mol Immunol* **30**:805–812.

Fuchs P, Breitling F, Dübel S, Seehaus T, Little M (1991) Targeting recombinant antibodies to the surface of *E coli*: fusion to a peptidoglycan associated lipoprotein. *Bio/Technology* **9**:1369–1372.

Fuchs P, Breitling F, Little M, Dübel S (1997) Primary structure and functional scFv antibody expression of an antibody against the human protooncogene c-myc. *Hybridoma* **16**:227–233.

Gandecha AR, Owen MR, Cockburn B, Whitelam GC (1992) Production and secretion of a bifunctional staphylococcal protein A antiphytochrome single-chain Fv fusion protein in *Escherichia coli*. *Gene* **122**:361–365.

Glockshuber R, Malia M, Pfitzinger I, Plückthun A (1990) A comparison of strategies to stabilize immunoglobulin Fv-fragments. *Biochemistry* **29**:1362–1367.

Glockshuber R, Schmidt T, Plückthun A (1992) The disulfide bonds in antibody variable domains: effects on stability, folding *in vitro*, and functional expression in *Escherichia coli*. *Biochemistry* **31**:1270–1279.

Gomi H, Hozumi T, Hattori S, Tagawa C, Kishimoto F, Bjorck L (1990) The gene sequence and some properties of protein H: a novel IgG-binding protein. *J Immunol* **144**:4046–4052.

Gotter S, Kipriyanov S, Haas C, Dübel S, Breitling F, Khazaie K, Schirrmacher V, Little M (1994) A *single-chain* antibody for coupling ligands to tumour cells infected with Newcastle disease virus. *Tumour Targeting* **1**:1–8.

Goward CR, Murphy JP, Atkinson T, Barstow DA (1990) Expression and purification of a truncated recombinant streptococcal protein G. *Biochem J* **267**:171–177.

Hardie G, van Regenmortel MHV (1975) Immunochemical studies of tobacco mosaic virus-I: refutation of the alleged homogeneous binding of purified antibody fragments. *Immunochemistry* **12**:903–908.

Harlow E, Lane D (1988) Antibodies. Cold Spring Harbor Laboratory, Cold Spring Harbor, NY.

Harris ELV, Angal S (1989) Protein purification methods: a practical approach. IRL Press Oxford, UK.

Harris RJ, Murnane AA, Utter SL, Wagner KL, Cox ET, Polastri GD, Helder JC, Sliwkowski MB (1993) Assessing genetic heterogeneity in production cell lines: detection by peptide mapping of a low level Tyr to Gln sequence variant in a recombinant antibody. *Biotechology NY* **11**:1293–1297.

Hasemann CA, Capra JD (1990) High-level production of a functional immunoglobulin heterodimer in a baculovirus expression system. *Proc Natl Acad Sci USA* **87**:3942–3946.

Hawkins RE, Russell SJ, Baier M, Winter G (1993) The contribution of contact and non-contact residues of antibody in the affinity of binding to antigen. The interaction of mutant D13 antibodies with lysozyme. *J Mol Biol* **234**:958–964.

Hengerer A, Hauck S, KöBlinger C, Wolf H and Dübel S (1990) Determination of phage antibody affinities to antigen by a microbalance sensor system (QCM). BioTechniques, *In Revision*.

Holvoet P, Laroche Y, Lijnen HR, Van-Cauwenberge R, Demarsin E, Brouwers E, Matthyssens G, Collen D (1991) Characterization of a chimeric plasminogen activator consisting of a single-chain Fv fragment derived from a fibrin fragment D-dimer-specific antibody and a truncated single-chain urokinase. *J Biol Chem* **266**:19717–19724.

Hopp TP, Gallis B, Prickett KS (1996) Metal-binding properties of a calcium-dependent monoclonal antibody. *Mol Immunol* **33**:601–608.

Horwitz AH, Chang CP, Better M, Hellstrom KE, Robinson RR (1988) Secretion of functional antibody and Fab fragment from yeast cells. *Proc Natl Acad Sci USA* **85**:8678–8682.

Hsu TA, Eiden JJ, Bourgarel P, Meo T, Betenbaugh MJ (1994) Effects of co-expressing chaperone BiP on functional antibody production in the baculovirus system. *Protein Expr Purif* **5**:595–603.

Hu P, Glasky MS, Yun A, Alauddin MM, Hornick JL, Khawli LA, Epstein AL (1995) A human-mouse chimeric Lym-1 monoclonal antibody with specificity for human lymphomas expressed in a baculovirus system. *Hum Antibodies Hybridomas* **6**:57–67.

Humphreys DP, Weir N, Lawson A, Mountain A, Lund Pa (1996) Coexpression of human protein disulphide isomerase (PDI) can increase the yield of an antibody Fab' fragment expressed in *Escherichia coli*. *FEBS Lett* **380**:194–197.

Huston JS, McCartney J, Tai MS, Mottola-Hartshorn C, Jin D, Warren F, Keck P, Oppermann H (1993) Medical applications of single-chain antibodies. Creative BioMolecules. Inc., Hopkinton, MA 01748. *Int Rev Immunol* **10**:195–217.

Issekutz AC (1983) Removal of gram-negative endotoxin from solutions by affinity chromatography. *J Immunol Methods* **61**:275–281.

Ito W, Iba Y, Kurosawa Y (1993) Effects of substitutions of closely related amino acids at the contact surface in an antigen-antibody complex on thermodynamic parameters. *J Biol Chem* **268**:16639–16647.

Jahn S, Roggenbuck D, Niemann B, Ward ES (1995) Expression of monovalent fragments derived from a human IgM autoantibody in *E. coli*: the input of the somatically mutated CDR1/CDR2 and of the CDR3 into antigen binding specificity. *Immunobiology* **193**:400–419.

Jarvis DL, Oker-Blom C, Summers MD (1990) Role of glycosylation in the transport of recombinant glycoproteins through the secretory pathway of lepid-opteran insect cells. *J Cell Biochem* **42**:181–191.

Johnson GA, Hansen TR, Austin KJ, Van, Kirk EA, Murdoch WJ (1995) Baculovirus-insect cell production of bioactive choriogonadotropin-immunoglobulin G heavy-chain fusion proteins in sheep. *Biol Reprod* **52**:68–73.

Jost CR, Kurucz I, Jacobus CM, Titus JA, George AJ, Segal DM (1994) Mammalian expression and secretion of functional single-chain Fv molecules. *J Biol Chem* **269**:26267–26273.

Jost CR, Titus JA, Kurucz I, Segal DM (1996) A single-chain bispecific Fv2 molecule produced in mammalian cells redirects lysis by activated CTL. *Mol Immunol* **33**:211–219.

Kabat EA, Wu TT, Reid-Miller M, Perry HM, Gottesman KS (1987) Sequences of proteins of immunological interest, US Department of Health And Human Services, US Government Printing Office, Washington, DC.

Kazemier B, de Haard H, Boender P, van Gemen B, Hoogenboom H (1996) Determination of active single chain antibody concentrations in crude periplasmic fractions. *J Immunol Methods* **194**:201–209.

Kelley RF, O'Connell MP, Carter P, Presta L, Eigenbrot C, Covarrubias M, Snedecor B, Bourell JH, Vetterlein D (1992) Antigen binding thermodynamics and antiproliferative effects of chimeric and humanized anti-p185HER2 antibody Fab fragments. *Biochemistry* **31**:5434–5441.

Keppel E, Schaller HC (1991) A 33 kDA protein with sequence homology to the 'laminin binding protein' is associated with the cytoskeleton in hydra and in mammalian cells. *J Cell Sci* **100**:789–797.

Keranen S, Penttila M (1995) Production of recombinant proteins in the filamentous fungus *Trichoderma reesei*. *Curr Opin Biotechnol* **6**:534–547.

King DJ, Byron OD, Mountain A, Weir N, Harvey A, Lawson AD, Proudfoot KA, Baldock D, Harding SE, Yarranton GT (1993) Expression, purification and characterization of B72.3 Fv fragments. *Biochem J* **290**:723–729.

King DJ, Turner A, Farnsworth AP, Adair JR, Owens RJ, Pedley RB, Baldock D, Proudfoot K A, Lawson AD, Beeley NR (1994) Improved tumor targeting with chemically cross-linked recombinant antibody fragments. *Cancer Res* **54**:6176–6185.

Kipriyanov S, Dübel S, Breitling F, Kontermann RE, Little M (1994) Recombinant single-chain Fv fragments carrying C-terminal cysteine residues: production of bivalent and biotinylated miniantibodies. *Mol Immun* **31**:1047–1058.

Kipriyanov S, Dübel S, Breitling F, Kontermann RE, Heymann S, Little M (1995a) Bacterial expression and refolding of single-chain Fv fragments with C-terminal cysteines. *Cell Biophys* **26**:187–204.

Kipriyanov SM, Breitling F, Little M, Dübel S (1995b) Single-chain antibody streptavidin fusions: tetrameric bifunctional scFv-complexes with biotin-binding activity and enhanced affinity to antigen. *Hum Antibod Hybridomas* **6**:93–101.

Kitchin K, Lin G, Shelver WL, Murtaugh MP, Pentel PR, Pond SM, Oberst JC, Humphrey JE, Smith JM, Flickinger MC (1995) Cloning, expression, and purification of an anti-desipramine single chain antibody in NS/O myeloma cells. *J Pharm Sci* **84**:1184–1189.

Kleymann G, Ostermeier C, Heitmann K, Haase W, Michel H (1995) Use of antibody fragments (Fv) in immunocytochemistry. *J Histochem Cytochem* **43**:607–614.

Knappik A, Plückthun A (1994) An improved affinity tag based on the FLAG peptide for the detection and purification of recombinant antibody fragments. *Biotechniques* **17**:754–761.

Knappik A, Plückthun A (1995) Engineered turns of a recombinant antibody improve its *in vivo* folding. *Protein-Eng* **8**:81–89.

Knappik A, Krebber C, Plückthun A (1993) The effect of folding catalysts on the *in vivo* folding process of different antibody fragment expressed in *Escherichia coli*. *Biotechnology NY* **11**:77–83.

Kneissel S, Queitsch I, Petersen G, Micheel B and Dübel S (1999) Epitope structures of antibodies against the major coat protein (g8p) of filamentous phage. J Mol Biol., *in revision*.

Kontermann RE, Liu Z, Schulze RA, Sommer KA, Queitsch I, Dübel S, Kipriyanov SM, Breitling F, Bautz EKF (1995) Characterization of the epitope recognised by a monoclonal antibody directed against the largest subunit of *Drosophila* RNA polymerase II. *Biol Chem Hoppe-Seyler* **376**:473–481.

Kortt AA, Malby RL, Caldwell JB, Gruen LC, Ivancic N, Lawrence MC, Howlett GJ, Webster RG, Hudson PJ, Colman PM (1994) Recombinant anti-sialidase single-chain variable fragments antibody: characterization, formation of dimer and higher-molecular-mass multimers and the solution of the crystal structure of single-chain variable fragment/sialidase complex. *Eur J Biochem* **221**:151–157.

Kretzschmar T, Aoustin L, Zingel O, Marangi M, Vonach B, Towbin H, Geiser M (1996) High-level expression in insect cells and purification of secreted monomeric single-chain Fv antibodies. *J Immunol Methods* **195**:93–101.

Lah M, Goldstraw A, White JF, Dolezal O, Malby R, Hudson PJ (1994) Phage surface presentation and secretion of antibody fragments using an adaptable phagemid vector. *Hum Antibodies Hybridomas* **5**:48–56.

Laroche Y, Demaeyer M, Stassen JM, Gansemans Y, Demarsin E, Matthyssens G, Collen D, Holvoet P (1991) Characterization of a recombinant single-chain molecule comprising the variable domains of a monoclonal antibody specific for human fibrin fragment D-dimer. *J Biol Chem* **266**:16343–16349.

Lethonen OP (1991) Immunoreactivity of solid phase hapten measured by a hapten binding plasmacytoma protein (ABPC24). *Mol Immunol* **18**:323–329.

Liu Z, Schneider-Mergener J, Martin A, Dandekar T, Bautz EKF, Dübel S (1999) Fine mapping of the antigen - antibody interaction of scFv215, a recombinant antibody inhibiting RNA polymerase II from *Drosophila melanogaster*. *J Molec Recognition*, in press.

Luo D, Mah N, Krantz M, Wilde K, Wishart D, Zhang Y, Jacobs F, Martin L (1995) Vl-linker-Vh orientation-dependent expression of single chain Fv-containing an engineered disulfide-stabilized bond in the framework regions. *J Biochem Tokyo* **118**:825–831.

MacCallum RM, Martin ACR, Thornton JT (1996) Antibody-antigen interactions: contact analysis and binding site topography. *J Mol Biol* **262**:732–745.

Mack M, Riethmuller G, Kufer P (1995) A small bispecific antibody construct expressed as a functional single-chain molecule with high tumor cell cytotoxicity. *Proc Natl Acad Sci USA* **92**:7021–7025.

MacKenzie CR, Sharma V, Brummell D, Bilous D, Dubuc G, Sadowska J, Young NM, Bundle DR, Narang SA (1994) Effect of Cλ-Cα domain switching of Fab' activity and yield in *E. coli*: Synthesis and expression of genes encoding two anti-carbohydrate Fab's. *Bio/Technology* **12**:390–395.

Maeda S (1989) Expression of foreign genes in insects using baculovirus vectors. *Annu Rev Entomol* **34**:351–372.

Matthews REF (1982) Classification and Nomenclature of Viruses. Karger Verlag, Basel.

Miceli RM, DeGraaf ME, Fischer HD (1994) Two-stage selection of sequences from a random phage display library delineates both core residues and permitted structural range within an epitope. *J Immunol Methods* **167**:279–287.

Milenic DE, Yokota T, Filpula DR, Finkelman MAJ, Dodd SW, Wood JF, Whitlow ML, Snoy P, Schlom J (1991) Construction, binding properties, metabolism and tumor targeting of a single-chain Fv derived from the pancarcinoma monoclonal antibody CC49. *Cancer Res* **51**:6363–6371.

Minobe S, Sato T, Tosa T, Chibata I (1983) Characteristics of immobilized histamine for pyrogen adsorption. *J Chromatogr* **252**:193–198.

Molloy PE, Graham BM, Cupit PM, Grant SD, Porter AJ, Cunningham C (1995) Expression and purification strategies for the production of single-chain antibody and T-cell receptor fragments in *E. coli*. *Mol Biotechnol* **4**:239–245.

Morton HC, Atkin JD, Owens RJ, Woof JM (1993) Purification and characterization of chimeric human IgA1 and IgA2 expressed in COS and Chinese hamster ovary cells. *J Immunol* **151**:4743–4752.

Nesbit M, Fu ZF, McDonald-Smith J, Steplewski Z, Curtis PJ (1992) Production of a functional monoclonal antibody recognizing human colorectal carcinoma cells from a baculovirus expression system. *J Immunol Methods* **151**:201–208.

Newton DL, Nicholls PJ, Rybak SM, Youle RJ (1994) Expression and characterization of recombinant human eosinophil-derived neurotoxin and eosinophil-derived neurotoxin-anti-transferrin receptor sFv. *J Biol. Chem* **269**:26739–26745.

Nicholls PJ, Johnson VG, Andrew SM, Hoogenboom HR, Raus JC, Youle RJ (1993) Characterization of single-chain antibody (sFv)-toxin fusion proteins produced *in vitro* in rabbit reticulocyte lysate. *J Biol chem* **268**:5302–5308.

Nilson BH, Solomon A, Bjorck L, Akerstrom B (1992) Protein L form *Peptostreptococcus magnus* binds to the kappa light chain variable domain. *J Biol Chem* **267**:2234–2239.

Nilson BH, Logdberg L, Kastern W, Bjorck L, Akerstrom B (1993) Purification of antibodies using protein l-binding framework structures in the light chain variable domain. *J Immunol Methods* **164**:33–40.

Nyyssonen E, Penttila M, Harkki A, Saloheimo A, Knowles JK, Keranen S (1993) Efficient production of antibody fragments by the filamentous fungus *Trichoderma reesei*. *Biotechnology NY* **11**:591–595.

Orfanoudakis G, Karim B, Bourel D, Weiss E (1993) Bacterially expressed Fabs of monoclonal antibodies neutralizing tumor necrosis factor alpha *in vitro* retain full binding and biological activity. *Mol Immunol* **30**:1519–1528.

Owen M, Gandecha A, Cockburn B, Whitelam G (1992) Synthesis of a functional anti-phytochrome single-chain Fv protein in transgenic tobacco. *Biotechnology NY* **10**:790–794.

Pack P, Kujau M, Schroeckh V, Knupfer U, Wenderoth R, Riesenberg D, Plückthun A (1993) Improved bivalent miniantibodies, with identical avidity as whole antibodies, produced by high cell density fermentation of *Escherichia coli*. *Biotechnology NY* **11**:1271–1277.

Page MJ, Sydenham MA (1991) High level expression of the humanized monoclonal antibody Campath-1H in Chinese hamster ovary cells. *Biotechnology NY* **9**:64–68.

Piccioli P, Di-Luzio A, Amann R, Schuligoi R, Surani MA, Donnerer J, Cattaneo A (1995) Neuroantibodies: extopic expression of a recombinant antisubstance P antibody in the central nervous system of transgenic mice. *Neuron* **15**:375–384.

Popov S, Hubbard JG, Ward ES (1996) A novel and efficient route for the isolation of antibodies that recognise T-cell receptor V alpha(s). *Mol Immunol* **33**:493–502.

Potter KN, Li YC, Capra JD (1994) The cross-reactive idiotopes recognized by the monoclonal antibodies 9G4 and LC1 are located in framework region 1 of two non-overlapping subsets of human VH4 family encoded antibodies. *Scand J Immunol* **40**:43–49.

Poul Ma, Cerutti M, Chaabihi H, Ticchioni M, Deramoudt FX, Bernard A, Devauchelle G, Kaczorek M, Lefranc MP (1995) Cassette baculovirus vectors for the production of chimeric humanized, or human antibodies in insect cells. *Eur J Immunol* **25**:2005–2009.

Proba K, Ge L, Plückthun A (1995) Functional antibody single-chain fragments from the cytoplasm of *Escherichia coli*: influence of thioredoxin reductase (TrxB). *Gene* **159**:203–207.

Proudfoot KA, Torrance C, Lawson AD, King DJ (1992) Purification of recombinant chimeric B72.3 Fab' and F(ab')2 using streptococcal protein G. *Protein Expr Purif* **3**:368–373.

Qi Y, Xiang J (1995) A genetically engineered single-gene-encoded anti-TAG72 chimeric antibody secreted from myeloma cells. *Hum Antibodies. Hybridomas* **6**:161–166.

Reis U, Blum B, von Specht BU, Domdey H, Collins J (1992) Antibody production in silkworm cells and silkworm larvae infected with a dual recombinant *Bombyx mori* nuclear polyhedrosis virus. *Biotechnology NY* **10**:910–912.

Reiter Y, Wright AF, Tonge DW, Pastan I (1996) Recombinant single-chain and disulfide-stabilized Fv-Immuntoxins that cause complete regression of a human colon cancer xenograft in nude mice. *Int J Cancer* **67**:113–123.

Rheinnecker M, Hardt C, Ilag LL, Kufer P, Gruber R, Hoess A, Lupas A, Rottenberger C, Plückthun A, Pack P (1996) Multivalent antibody fragments with high functional affinity for a tumor-associated carbohydrate antigen. *J Immunol* **157**:2989–2997.

Ridder R, Geisse S, Kleuser B, Kawalleck P, Gram HA (1995a) COS-cell-based system for rapid production and quantification of scFv::IgC kappa antibody fragments. *Gene* **166**:273–276.

Ridder R, Schmitz R, Legay F, Gram H (1995b) Generation of rabbit monoclonal antibody fragments from a combinatorial phage display library and their production in the yeast *Pichia pastoris*. *Bio/Technology* **13**:255–260.

Roggenbuck D, Konig H, Niemann B, Schoenherr G, Jahn S, Porstmann T (1994) Real-time biospecific interaction analysis of a natural human polyreactive monoclonal IgM antibody and its Fab and scFv fragments with several antigens. *Scand J Immunol* **40**:64–70.

Ross CN, Turner N, Savage P, Cashman SJ, Spooner RA, Pusey CD (1996) A single-chain Fv reactive with the Goodpasture antigen. *Lab Invest* **74**:1051–1059.

Rosso MN, Schouten A, Roosien J, Borst-Vrenssen T, Hussey RS, Gommers FJ, Bakker J, Schots A, Abad P (1996) Expression and functional characterization of a single-chain Fv antibody directed against secretions involved in plant nematode infection process. *Biochem Biophys Res Commun* **220**:255–263.

Sambrook J, Fritsch EF, Maniatis T (1989) Molecular cloning, a laboratory manual. Cold Spring Harbor Laboratory Press, Cold Spring Harbor, NY.

Sasso EH, Silverman GJ, Mannik M (1991) Human IgA and IgG F(ab')2 that bind to staphylococcal protein A belong to the VHIII subgroup. *J Immunol* **147**:1877–1883.

Sawyer JR, Schlom J, Kashmiri SV (1994) The effects of induction conditions on production of a soluble anti-tumor scFv in *Escherichia coli*. *Protein Eng* **7**:1401–1406.

Schiweck W, Skerra A (1995) Fermenter production of an artificial Fab fragment, rationally designed for the antigen cystatin, and its optimized crystallization through constant domain shuttling. *Proteins* **23**:561–565.

Schmidt TG, Skerra A (1993) The random peptide library-assisted engineering of a C-terminal affinity peptide, useful for the detection and purification of a functional Ig Fv fragment. *Protein Eng* **6**:109–122.

Schmidt TG, Koepke J, Frank R, Skerra A (1996) Molecular interaction between the Strep-tag affinity peptide and its cognate target, streptavidin. *J Mol Biol* **255**:753–766.

Schouten A, Roosien J, van-Engelen FA, de Jong GA, Borst-Vrenssen AW, Zilverentant JF, Bosch D, Stiekema WJ, Gommers FJ, Schots A, Bakker J (1996) the C-terminal KDEL sequence increases the expression level of a single-chain antibody designed to be targeted to both the cytosol and the secretory pathway in transgenic tobacco. *Plant Mol Biol* **30**:781–793.

Schulze RA, Kontermann RE, Queitsch I, Dübel S, Bautz EKF (1994) Thiophilic adsorption chromatography of single-chain antibody fragments. *Anal Biochem* **220**:212–214.

Serhir B, Dubreuil D, Higgins R, Jacques M (1995) Purification and characterization of a 52-kilodalton immunoglobulin G-binding protein from *Streptococcus suis* capsular type 2. *J Bacteriol* **177**:3830–3836.

Shelver WL, Keyler DE, Lin G, Murtaugh MP, Flickinger MC, Ross CA, Pentel PR (1996) Effects of recombinant drug-specific single-chain antibody Fv fragment on [3H]-desipramine distribution in rats. *Biochem Pharmacol* **51**:531–537.

Shu L, Qi CF, Schlom J, Kashmiri SV (1993) Secretion of a single-gene-encoded immunoglobulin from myeloma cells. *Proc Natl Acad Sci USA* **90**:7995–7999.

Skerra A (1994) A general vector, pASK84, for cloning, bacterial production, and single-step purification of antibody Fab fragments. *Gene* **141**:79–84.

Skerra A, Plückthun A (1988) Assembly of a functional immunoglobulin Fv fragment in *Escherichia coli*. *Science* **240**:1038–1051.

Skerra A, Plückthun A (1991) Secretion and *in vivo* folding of the Fab' fragment of the antibody McPC603 in *Escherichia coli*: influence of disulphides and cis-prolines. *Protein Eng* **4**:971–979.

Skerra A, Pfitzinger I, Plückthun A (1991) The functional expression of antibody Fv fragments in *Escherichia coli*: improved vectors and a generally applicable purification technique. *Biotechnology NY* **9**:273–278.

Sohi MK, Wan T, Sutton BJ, Atkinson T, Atkinson MA, Murphy JP, Bottomley SP, Gore MG (1995) Crystallization and X-ray analysis of a single fab binding domain from protein L of *Peptostreptococcus magnus*. *Proteins* **23**:610–612.

Somerville JE, Goshorn SC, Fell HP, Darveau RP (1994) Bacterial aspects associated with the expression of a single-chain antibody fragment in *Escherichia coli*. *Appl Microbiol Biotechnol* **42**:595–603.

Song Z, Cai Y, Song D, Xu J, Yuan H, Wang L, Zhu X, Lin H, Breitling F, Dübel S (1997) Primary structure and functional expression of heavy- and light-chain variable region genes of a monoclonal antibody specific for human fibrin. *Hybridoma* **16**:235–241.

Spence C, Nachman M, Gately MK, Kreitman FJ, Pastan L, Bailon P (1993) Affinity purification and characterization of anti-Tac(Fv)-C3-PE38KDEL: A highly potent cytotoxic agent specific to cells bearing IL-2 receptors. *Bioconjug Chem* **40**:63–68.

Stemmer WPC, Morris SK, Kautzer CK, Wilson BS (1993) Increased antibody expression from *E. coli* through wobble-base library mutagenesis by enzymatic inverse PCR. *Gene* **123**:1–7.

Sulkowski E (1985) Immobilised metal affinity chromatography. *Trends Biotechnol* **3**:1–7.

Tai MS, Mudgett Hunter M, Levinson D, Wu GM, Haber E, Oppermann H, Huston JS (1990) A bifunctional fusion protein containing Fc-binding fragment B of staphylococcal protein A amino terminal to antidigoxin single-chain Fv. *Biochemistry* **29**:8024–8030.

Talmadge KW, Siebert CJ (1989) Efficient endotoxin removal with a new sanitizable affinity column: Affi-Prep Polymyxin. *J Chromatogr* **476**:175–185.

Thielemans KM (1995) Immunotheraphy with bispecific antibodies. *Verh K Acad Geneeskd Belg* **57**:229–247.

Tsumoto K, Nakaoki Y, Ueda Y, Ogasahara K, Yutani K, Watanabe K, Kumagai I (1994) Effect of the order of antibody variable regions on the expression of the single-chain HyHEL10Fv fragment in *E. coli* and the thermodynamic analysis of its antigen-binding properties. *Biochem Biophys Res Commun* **201**:546–551.

Ueda Y, Tsumoto K, Watanabe K, Kumagai I (1993) Synthesis and expression of a DNA encoding the Fv domain of an anti-lysozyme monoclonal antibody, HyHEL10, in *Streptomyces lividans*. *Gene* **129**:129–134.

Ulrich HD, Platien PA, Yang PL, Romesber FE, Schultz PG (1995) Expression studies of catalytic antibodies. *Proc Natl Acad Sci USA* **92**:11907–11911.

Underwood PA (1985) Practical considerations of the ability of monoclonal antibodies to detect antigenic difference between closely related variants. *J Immunol Methods* **85**:309–323.

Voss S, Skerra A (1997) Mutagenesis of a flexible loop in streptavidin leads to higher affinity for the Strep-tag II peptide and improved performance in recombinant protein purification. *Protein-Eng* **10**:975–82.

Ward ES, Güssow D, Griffiths AD, Jones PT, Winter G (1989) Binding activites of a repertoir of a single immunoglobulin variable domains secreted from *Escherichia coli*. *Nature* **341**:544–546.

Ward VK, Kreissig SB, Hammock BD, Choudary PV (1995) Generation of an expression library in the baculovirus expression vector system. *J Virol Methods* **53**:263–272.

Werge TM, Bradbury A, Di Luzio A, Cattaneo A (1992) A recombinant cell line expressing a form of the Y13-259 anti-p21ras antibody which binds protein A and may be produced as ascites. *Oncogene* **7**:1033–1035.

Whitlow M, Bell BA, Feng S-L, Fipula D, Hardman KD, Hubert SL, Rollence ML; Wood JF, Schott ME, Milenic DE, Yokota T, Schlom J (1993) An improved linker for single-chain Fv with reduced aggregation and enhanced proteolytic stability. *Protein Eng* **6**:989–995.

Wilson BS, Kautzer CR, Antelman DE (1994) Increased protein expression through improved ribosome-binding sites obtained by library mutagenesis. *Biotechniques* **17**:944–953.

Wu AM, Williams LE, Wong JYC, Shively JE, Raubitschek AA (1996) Genetically engineered anti-caroinembryonic antigen (CEA) antibodies and fragments: preclinical and clinical radioimaging studies. Proceedings of the GBF- Symposiums Antibody Technology and Applications in Health and Environment, Braunscheweig, Sept. 1996.

Wu XC, Ng SC, Near RI, Wong WL (1993) Efficient production of a functional single-chain antidigoxin antibody via an engineered *Bacillus subtilis* expression-secretion system, *Biotechnology NY* **11**:71–76.

Yokota T, Milenic DE, Whitlow DE, Whitlow M, Schlom J (1992) Rapid tumor penetration of a single-chain Fv and comparison with other immunoglobulin forms. *Cancer Res* **52**:3402–3408.

Zewe M, Rybak SM, Dübel S, Coy JF, Welschof M, Newton DL, Little M (1997) Cloning and cytotoxicity of a human pancreatic RNase immunofusion. *Immunotechnology* **3**:127–136.

Zu Putlitz J, Kubasek WL, Duchene M, Marget M, von Specht BU, Domdey H (1990) Antibody production in baculovirus-infected insect cells. *Biotechnology NY* **8**:651–654.

Index